Tumor Deposits

Sulen Sarioglu

Tumor Deposits

Mechanism, Morphology and Prognostic Implications

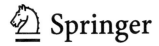 Springer

Sulen Sarioglu
Department of Pathology
Dokuz Eylul University
Inciralti Balcova/Izmir
Turkey

ISBN 978-3-319-88624-4   ISBN 978-3-319-68582-3   (eBook)
https://doi.org/10.1007/978-3-319-68582-3

© Springer International Publishing AG 2018
Softcover re-print of the Hardcover 1st edition 2018
This work is subject to copyright. All rights are reserved by the Publisher, whether the whole or part of the material is concerned, specifically the rights of translation, reprinting, reuse of illustrations, recitation, broadcasting, reproduction on microfilms or in any other physical way, and transmission or information storage and retrieval, electronic adaptation, computer software, or by similar or dissimilar methodology now known or hereafter developed.
The use of general descriptive names, registered names, trademarks, service marks, etc. in this publication does not imply, even in the absence of a specific statement, that such names are exempt from the relevant protective laws and regulations and therefore free for general use.
The publisher, the authors and the editors are safe to assume that the advice and information in this book are believed to be true and accurate at the date of publication. Neither the publisher nor the authors or the editors give a warranty, express or implied, with respect to the material contained herein or for any errors or omissions that may have been made. The publisher remains neutral with regard to jurisdictional claims in published maps and institutional affiliations.

Printed on acid-free paper

This Springer imprint is published by Springer Nature
The registered company is Springer International Publishing AG
The registered company address is: Gewerbestrasse 11, 6330 Cham, Switzerland

To
My teachers

To
Dokuz Eylul University Colorectal Oncology
Group and Head and Neck Oncology Group
For constant flow of scientific information for
management of patients

To my father and mother

To my spouse
For his support and patience

Preface

Some of the valuable, potentially cornerstone information in medicine may be overlooked and this seems to be multifactorial and the mechanisms seem to be time dependent. Previously, the reason for this negligence may have been related to the difficulties of publication and distribution. Furthermore, some observations were hard to prove due to lack of suitable scientific methods. Recently, the main reason may be excessive information.

Two interesting hypotheses that were forgotten or underestimated for many decades but flourishing recently in cancer growth and dissemination are the tendency of anaerobic glycolysis and hunger for glucose of the tumor cells by Dr. Otto Warburg and *seed and soil* hypothesis by Sir James Paget.

Like these observations, in 1935, Gabriel WB, Dukes CE, and Bussey HJR observed and described the tumor deposits in colorectal carcinomas. These lesions attracted the most attention in this organ system and were included in the TNM classification after many decades, in the fifth edition in 1997, and with each update, the classification and description of the lesion changed. Nevertheless, the inclusion in TNM classification at least in one organ system legalized the tumor deposits as specific lesions leading to further research in different organ systems.

Gastric, esophageal, head, and neck carcinomas are the ones with information about the morphology, mechanism, and prognostic value of tumor deposits as well as the colorectal carcinoma cases; however, the studies are still few in number and there are no studies in many types of carcinomas like one of the most frequent carcinomas, the breast carcinomas.

This book focuses on the mechanisms of metastasis and tumor deposit formation. Tumor deposits seem to be the result of extramural perivascular and/or perineural migratory metastasis mechanisms as well as lymphatic/vascular extravasations, a series of morphological and molecular events different from the classical pathways of metastasis. The understanding of these mechanisms may lead to targeted therapies preventing this type of tumor dissemination. The most important step for this goal is recognition of this type of spread as a basic mechanism of metastasis.

In this book, information about the importance of tumor deposits in different organs was presented. The association of tumor deposits and poor prognosis is striking in all organs.

Furthermore, the frequent association of peritoneal carcinomatosis and tumor deposits was highlighted, and the possible relationships of these lesions were discussed.

The book is intended to provide an overview of the available information about tumor deposits in the literature and lay emphasis on the requirement of further research in this field, a major mechanism of tumor dissemination.

The different terminology used in different articles, different morphological criteria applied for the diagnosis of tumor deposits, and even different methods of macroscopic evaluation made it hard to prepare the book. All these aspects were discussed in the book and the lesions were presented with many microscopic images.

I hope this book will help to keep the tumor deposits in focus of oncological research and be helpful for the readers dealing with pathology and oncology, finally helping to prolong the disease-free or overall survival of the patients.

Izmir, Turkey   Sulen Sarioglu

Acknowledgment

I want to thank Springer and Dr. Inga von Behrens for encouraging me to write this book. I would not have written the book if she had not made a proposal. I'm also thankful to Mr. Prakash Jagannathan during the process of writing the book. I received kind reminders from him and probably I would not be able to finish the project in time without them. Many thanks to the team performing the reduction of the text; they were excellent in helping an author who is not a native English speaker.

Many thanks to all my teachers in medicine and pathology, all my colleagues and students, and all my patients; they taught me to observe, question, and discuss.

Contents

Mechanisms of Metastasis

Metastasis is an ancient Greek word which means displacement. It is a word coined with malignant tumor dissemination, the displacement of cells which have malignant behavioral potential, to travel and home to another tissue. The term was introduced to the medical literature by Joseph-Claude-Anthelme Récamier (6 November 1774–28 June 1852), a French gynecologist (Weber 2013). Understanding the mechanisms, early and correct diagnosis, and optional treatment of metastasis are of utmost importance in oncological patient management as metastasis is the main prognostic factor in malignant tumors.

Progression of malignant tumors is a multistep process. Malignant tumors are made up of monoclonal but heterogeneous cells. Tumors are derived from a single cell with a driver mutation, so all the tumors are monoclonal. Only one driver mutation is not enough for progression of a malignant tumor; however, cells with a driver mutation are prone to the accumulation of mutations leading to malignant cell transformation. The mutations following the driver mutation may be different in different cells originating from the first mutated cell, and this leads to a heterogeneous population and finally intratumoral heterogeneity.

Healthy cells have many properties; they perform exactly the excellent behaviors for the well-being of the organism they are part of. This type of situation is named as "homeostasis," and this situation requires innumerable functions, and probably an unknown amount is still beyond our scientific knowledge.

The differences between a cell at homeostasis and malignant tumor cell are numerous. The first step to discuss the mechanisms of metastasis may be starting with a summary of normal cellular structure and function compared with a neoplastic cell. However, this will not be satisfactory as the tumor tissue, including neoplastic cells, tumor stroma with vasculature, and tumor reactive inflammatory component, acts in complex interaction during tumor progression; ignoring these important contributors will result in an underestimation of the complexity of neoplastic transformation and behavior. So basically, this chapter will first focus on the differences between a cell at homeostasis and a neoplastic cell, followed by the changes in tumor stroma and immune response.

© Springer International Publishing AG 2018
S. Sarioglu, *Tumor Deposits*, https://doi.org/10.1007/978-3-319-68582-3_1

Metastasis will be the following issue of this chapter as it is in tumor progression. Invasion, loss of adhesion (detachment), dissemination through different routes and traveling (migration), homing (adhesion), and colonization along with the formation of tumor stroma will be discussed.

Normal Tissue Versus Malignant Neoplasia

Neoplasms share many structural and functional features with normal tissues and cells. Neoplasms may be divided into two groups:

- Benign neoplasms
- Malignant neoplasms

This book and chapter focus on "metastasis," a feature of malignant neoplasms. The specific features of benign neoplasms are not targeted and will not be discussed in detail.

The neoplasms are classified according to their tissue or cellular origin. Most of the research about metastasis is focused on tumors arising from the epithelium, which covers all the surfaces of the body including the glandular structures. Although sarcomas have metastatic potential, the chapter will focus mainly on the behavior of the carcinomas, the most common type of tumor. However, at some relevant points, different type of neoplasms will be included, like malignant melanomas.

In 2000, Hanahan and Weinberg listed "hallmarks" of cancer, and then the list was expanded in 2012 including the following (Hanahan and Weinberg 2000, 2011); this very precise list summarizes the features of the cancer that are different from the normal cells and tissues:

- Self-sufficiency in growth signals
- Insensitivity to growth-inhibitory (antigrowth) signals
- Evasion of apoptosis
- Limitless replicative potential
- Sustained angiogenesis
- Tissue invasion
- Metastasis
- Reprogramming of the energy metabolism
- Evading immune response
- Tumor microenvironment

Malignant tumors have different characteristics from normal cells:

Gross Morphology: Malignant tumors make up a mass replacing the normal tissues and structures. They may be polypoid, ulcerated, or infiltrative, creating irregular borders with the surrounding normal tissue. Hemorrhage and necrosis may be observed. Tumors may destroy, replace, push, and distort the normal tissues and impair normal function. They may lead to perforation, bleeding, or loss of function.

Light Microscopy: Normal tissue cells have similar nuclear and cytoplasmic features with each other if they are of the same type. Epithelial cells grow in an orderly fashion, keeping up with the "polarity"; the basal epithelial cells are small with higher nucleocytoplasmic ratio, and as they replace to parabasal cells, they get a little smaller nuclei and larger cytoplasm. Nuclear-to-cytoplasmic ratio is about ¼ to 1/6. In contrast, malignant cells are pleomorphic; cells have different sizes and shapes with a nuclear-to-cytoplasmic ratio of 1/1. Nuclear membranes are frequently irregular and nuclei stain more purple (*hyperchromatism*). Furthermore, malignant cells sometimes strongly resemble the cells they are derived from, in this case they are well differentiated but sometimes it gets hard to recognize their cell or tissue of origin, and in this case, they are poorly differentiated, and this loss of differentiation is named as *anaplasia*. This reflects a differentiation at a more primitive level (Fig. 1.1).

The cellular changes are associated with architectural changes in malignant neoplasia. Considering carcinomas arising from glandular cells, it may be hard to see any glandular structures, if the case is poorly differentiated or high grade. In well-differentiated carcinomas, *complex-cribriform glandular pattern* and nuclear atypia are the main features for diagnosis, along with invasion. Histopathological diagnosis of carcinoma requires identification of invasion in most of the cases.

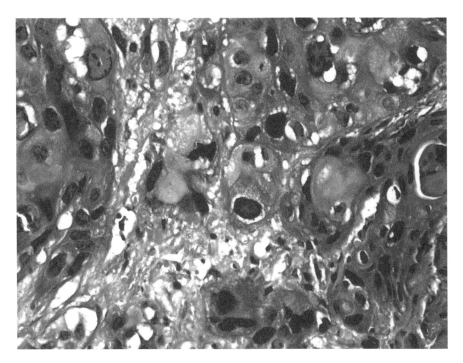

Fig. 1.1 Anaplastic malignant cells from a high-grade squamous cell carcinoma; cellular pleomorphism, anisonucleosis, hyperchromasia, chromatin distribution irregularity, and distinct nucleoli are seen (H&E, original magnification ×40)

Invasion is the growth of the neoplastic cells into the stroma, losing their connections at least partially with their neighbor epithelial cells, destroying and getting beyond the basement membrane. Invasion may be as single cells or clusters of cells.

Mitotic activity is increased in tumors, but high mitotic activity is not diagnostic for neoplasia. However atypical mitosis is a feature of neoplasia, and it can be recognized by disproportioned distribution of the chromosomes, and instead of the bipolar spindles seen in normal cells, tripolar or quadripolar spindles are seen (Fig. 1.2).

Tumor stroma and vasculature are also different from normal tissue. Tumor stroma has a specific type of fibrotic structure which is also active in tumor growth and named as *desmoplasia* (Sis et al. 2004; Unlu et al. 2013). Angiogenesis is a feature that is required for tumor growth, and it is a feature of malignant tumors and is a poor prognostic factor (Sökmen et al. 2001a, b). Angiogenesis may not be enough for sufficient supplies like nutrients and oxygen for the tumor, and necrosis is a frequently identified feature of malignant tumors which is also a prognostic factor in some types of carcinomas (Gurel et al. 2016).

The morphological features of the tumors are the reflection of genetic and epigenetic changes starting from the preinvasive tumor phase and ensuing in a multistep pattern (Sarioğlu et al. 2001; Sengiz et al. 2004); these complex mechanisms will be discussed in the following pages.

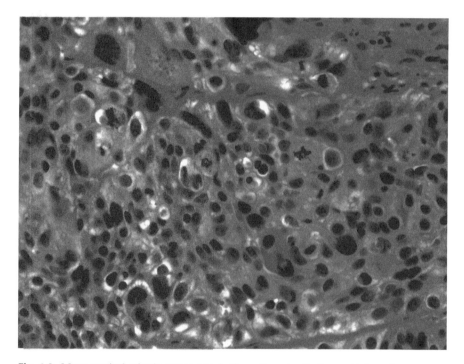

Fig. 1.2 Many atypical mitosis among anaplastic malignant cells from a high-grade squamous cell carcinoma (H&E, original magnification ×40)

Molecular and Genetic Features

Normal cells have an ideal proliferative capacity; they proliferate precisely as much as necessary and finish the proliferative activity when the stimulus is over. This is balanced with two sets of genes which induce or suppress proliferation. Unfortunately, these are named coined with neoplasia, even under normal conditions. *Tumor suppressor genes* are the ones which suppress proliferation.

The ones that induce cell proliferation are named as proto-oncogenes in normal cells. After mutation, they may be expressed in an uncontrolled manner or overexpression, and/or resistance to degradation may be seen, and these result in increased cellular proliferation. Mutation in only one allele is enough for increased proliferation in many cases. High proliferative activity results in uncontrolled DNA replication, and this increases the risk of additional mutations. Types of oncogenes may be listed as follows:

- Growth factors: e.g., transforming growth factor alpha (TGF-α) and platelet-derived growth factor (PDGF).
- Growth factor receptors: tyrosine kinase receptors seem to be the most important groups, e.g., *ERBB1* point mutations, *ERBB2* amplification, *EML4-ALK* fusion gene, and mutation or amplification of epidermal growth factor receptor (EGFR) (Demiral et al. 2004).
- Downstream components of the tyrosine kinase pathway: *RAS*, *BRAF*, and *PI3K*.
- Alterations in nonreceptor tyrosine kinases.
- Transcription factors: example, *MYC*, *MYB*, *JUN*, and *FOS*.
- Cyclins and cyclin-dependent kinases.

The genes that suppress cell proliferation or act as brakes for proliferation are the tumor suppressor genes. These genes also check the integrity of DNA structure and push the brakes of proliferation till this problem is solved. Loss of two alleles is required for the loss of the tumor suppressor functions; however, allele insufficiency and other rare exceptions should be kept in mind. Types of tumor suppressor genes may be listed as follows:'

- Inhibitors of mitogenic signaling pathways: examples are *APC*, *NF1*, *NF2*, *PTEN*, and *SMAD2*.
- Inhibitors of cell cycle progression: an example is retinoblastoma *(Rb)*.
- Inhibitors of metabolism and angiogenesis: examples are *VHL* and *STK11*.
- Inhibitors of invasion and metastasis: an example is *CDH1* encoding E-cadherin.
- Genetic stability: an example is *p53*.
- DNA repair genes: examples are *BRCA1*, *BRCA2*, *MLH1*, *MSH2*, *MSH6*, and *PMS2* (Kumar V et al. 2015; Hanahan D 2011).

Genomic Instability

Normal cells have the ability to solve problems of DNA damage, by multiple mechanisms:

- The activities of the DNA repair genes
- Apoptosis if the damage is unrepairable
- Oncogene-induced senescence
- Immune surveillance

Loss of the DNA repair mechanisms is important in mutations to get fixed, transferred to next cell generations following successful cell division. The Nobel Prizes in Chemistry were awarded to three scientists for their discoveries for the mechanistic mechanisms of the DNA repair, namely, Tomas Lindahl (Lindahl 2013), Paul Modrich (Modrich 1994), and Aziz Sancar.

Mismatch repair genes function during replication to prevent any replication errors or misplacement of a nucleotide in particular. The mutation or loss of these genes, including *MLH1*, *MSH2*, *MSH6*, and *PMS2*, which are important in colorectal carcinomas, is important in carcinogenesis and results in microsatellite instability. Microsatellites are one to six nucleotides distributed in the DNA, and they are same for every cell of an individual, but there are differences between each person, so the matching of the microsatellites is used for identification of persons or paternity tests in forensic medicine. However, the mutations or losses of mismatch repair genes result in other mutations which may lead to cancer development. Genetic mismatch repair gene mutations lead to Lynch syndrome with risk of early right-sided colorectal carcinoma and endometrial, ovarian, stomach, small bowel, and urothelial carcinomas (Lynch and Smyrk 1996, Modrich P 1994).

Cross-linking of pyrimidine residues prevents DNA replication. In normal cells, this type of damage is solved by nucleotide excision system which includes many enzymes. Ultraviolet light is the most important factor that leads to this type of DNA damage, and if there are mutations of nucleotide excision system genes, the patient develops many skin tumors at the sun-exposed areas, and this disease is named as "xeroderma pigmentosum" (Sancar 1996).

There are multiple cancer syndromes with inherited mutations which may also be acquired during carcinogenesis.

Metabolic Alterations

Otto Warburg (Nobel Physiology and Medicine Prize laureate, 1931) presented the switch of the carcinoma cells to *aerobic glycolysis* even in case of sufficient vascular supply. The glucose hunger of the carcinoma cells is well known, and positron emission tomography (PET) which is extensively used for primary and metastatic cancer detection operates with this information, using radiolabeled F-fluorodeoxyglucose. This type of metabolism is not mutually exclusive for malignant cells, and again they are a function of normal cells during growth phase;

however, it is permanent in carcinoma cells. This metabolic change helps the cells to grow without oxygen, and the breakdown components are used in building of the multiplying tumor cells. This metabolic change may be related to multiple factors; for example, it may be induced by proto-oncogene *MYC* in growing cells, while the cause may be the oncogene *MYC* in carcinomas.

Angiogenesis is a prerequisite for cancer progression. Although increased vascular structures are found to be a poor prognostic marker in different series (Sökmen et al. 2001a, b), tumor hypoxia is also a poor prognostic factor (Cooper et al. 2003). It seems angiogenesis is required for tumor growth, but tumor metabolic changes, as suggested by Otto Warburg many decades ago, alter the tumor behavior.

Limitless Replicative Potential

In relation to limitless replicative potential, three scientists were awarded the Physiology or Medicine Nobel Prize in 2009: Elizabeth H. Blackburn, Carol W. Greider, and Jack W. Szostak. Their studies on the role of the telomeres and telomerase enzyme in protection of the DNA brought them the award (Greider and Blackburn 1985, 1987).

Telomeres are found at the ends of the chromosomes and are made of six nucleotides: TTTAGG. They prevent the end-to-end fusion of the chromosomes and help keep DNA integrity. Telomeres get shorter with the divisions of the somatic cells resulting in end replication problem. Under these conditions, the checkpoints of the cells, including p53, lead the cells to replicative senescence, irreversible loss of cellular proliferative capacity. However these cells do not replicate, but they don't die for a prolonged period either. Rarely the fusion of the end points with distinctly shortened telomeres may result in genomic instability with increased risk for mutation.

Stem cells have telomerase activity; this enzyme that allows unlimited replicative potential counteracts with telomere shortening. Either telomerase activity or alternative telomere lengthening (ATL) is a feature of malignant cells; the latter is more frequently activated in mesenchymal tumors and is associated with poor prognosis. Telomerase is a reverse transcriptase enzyme made up of RNA and protein components with the ability to use the RNA as a template in order to extend DNA 3' ends (Dikmen et al. 2009, Millet and Makovets 2016). Another mechanism for survival was suggested to be chromosome VIII aneuploidy, for overcoming telomere insufficiency (Millet and Makovets 2016).

Telomerase template antagonists are among the targets of tumor treatment, as one of the features of tumor cells is unlimited replicative potential (Dikmen et al. 2009).

Angiogenesis, Vasculogenesis, Vascular Co-option, Lymphangiogenesis, and Neoneurogenesis

Angiogenesis (sprouting) and vasculogenesis (tubule formation) are active during embryogenesis and temporarily activated during wound healing as well as menstrual cycle in adults. Angiogenic switch is turned on during tumor progression.

The mechanism of *neoangiogenesis* induced by tumor cells through soluble factors during tumor progression was introduced in the 1970s by Folkman et al. (1971). This led to the discoveries of factors like vascular endothelial growth factors and their receptors influencing angiogenesis as well as the inhibitors of angiogenesis.

Vascular endothelial growth factor, which is induced by hypoxia and oncogenes like *Ras* and *Myc*, and its receptors are important in this process. Bone marrow-derived vascular progenitor cells also contribute to angiogenesis, differentiating into endothelial cells and pericytes (Hanahan D 2011).

Although angiogenesis is accepted as a prerequisite for tumor progression, the failures of antiangiogenic therapies in tumor control in metastatic diseases raised questions about other sources of blood (Donnem et al. 2013). The utilization of the preexisting vasculature may be an alternative, and this is named as vessel co-option. In a series by Bridgeman et al. 2017, 164 lung metastatic lesions from breast, colorectal, and renal carcinomas were evaluated and grouped according to the histological growth patterns, and different mechanisms for vessel co-option were suggested, supported by a set of excellent immunohistochemistry evaluations, as follows:

- Alveolar pattern: co-option with alveolar capillaries
- Interstitial: co-option with alveolar capillaries
- Perivascular cuffing: co-option with larger vessels
- Pushing: mechanism unknown for vessel co-option

In this series, 80% of the cases were suggested to have vascular co-option. Vessel co-option and angiogenesis may be associated, and co-opted vessels may be the center for angiogenesis.

Another very important mechanism during tumor progression is *lymphangiogenesis*, and following the proper identification of lymphatics by specific antibodies like LYVE1 and podoplanin, it was proposed as a prognostic factor in different types of carcinomas.

Like neoangiogenesis and lymphangiogenesis, there is some evidence for *neo-neurogenesis* during tumor progression. The perineural invasion is a basic route for tumor dissemination (Fig. 1.3). Nerve endings were identified inside the tumor tissue, and even neoformation of axon was presented in prostatic carcinoma. The interaction of nerves and neoplastic cells is not limited to invasion of the neural structures by the tumor cells, but there seems to be a continuous interaction between the nervous system and the tumors through neurotransmitters. Unfortunately not all of the neurotransmitters act in the direction of tumor suppression (Mancino et al. 2011).

Autophagy

Cells may eat their contents as well as the nutrients they achieve from the intercellular area, and this self-feeding process is named as *autophagy*, a cellular function which is induced in different conditions like hypoxia and/or deficiency of the nutrients and/or

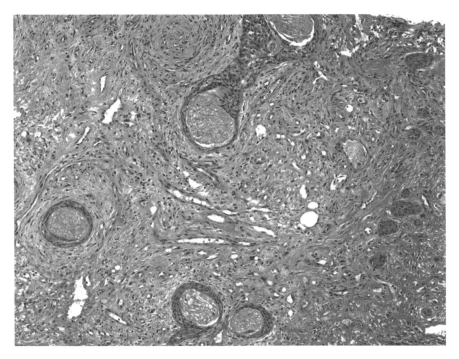

Fig. 1.3 Perineural invasion by squamous cell carcinoma (H&E, original magnification ×10)

growth factors, regulated both at the transcription and posttranscription level. The importance of this mechanism is crowned in 2016 by the Physiology or Medicine Nobel Prize which was attributed to Yoshinori Ohsumi for his work on the mechanisms of autophagy. The autophagy signals and lysosomal function are connected.

Many steps of carcinogenesis and metastasis are related to autophagy.

Autophagic flux may be divided into stages:

- Initiation, elongation, and closure
- Maturation
- Fusion with lysosomes
- Breakdown and release of macromolecules back to the cytosol

Multiple markers may be used for revealing the autophagic flux. Beclin-1 and microtubule-associated light chain (LC3) expressions are markers of autophagosome formation. mTOR is a master regulator of autophagy, and there is an inverse relation between autophagy induction and mTOR activation. p62 is a marker of autophagic degradation (Kabeya et al. 2000, Pattingre et al. 2008, Sahni et al. 2014, Katsuragi et al. 2015, Lee and Lee 2016, Wu et al. 2017).

The regulation of autophagic influx is complex and induced by reduced nutrient availability. The findings are in favor of the relationship of increased autophagy markers with aggressive tumor behavior, metastasis, and poor prognosis. The effects of autophagy have been demonstrated at multiple stages in cancer progression including regulation of EMT, invasion, migration, survival of distributed and circulating tumor cells, promotion of stem-like properties, as well as drug resistance in tumor cells (Mowers et al. 2016).

Apoptosis, Necroptosis, and Anoikis

Apoptosis

John Foxton Ross Kerr, an Australian pathologist, first described the ultrastructural changes in programmed cell death and then proposed the terminology of *apoptosis* in 1972 (Kerr et al. 1972). Sydney Brenner, H. Robert Horvitz, and John E. Sulston received the Nobel Prize for their discoveries concerning genetic regulation of organ development and programmed cell death in 2002.

Apoptosis is a word in Greek, which means falling of the leaves from trees or dropping of the petals from flowers. This is a basic mechanism in homeostasis, and it plays important roles during embryonic development. Apoptosis has distinct morphological and molecular features due to activated DNA endonucleases, fragmenting the DNA and giving rise to apoptotic bodies made of small condensed DNA and cytoplasmic fragments (Fig. 1.4). Apoptotic bodies do not induce inflammation but

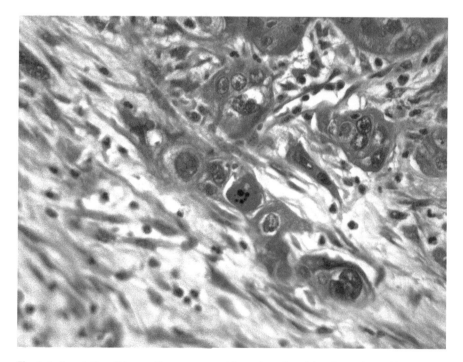

Fig. 1.4 Apoptotic cell in a malignant tumor with condensed nuclei and cytoplasm. Although the apoptotic pathways are corrupted during carcinogenesis and decreased apoptosis is expected in neoplasia, many apoptotic cells are seen in neoplastic tissue. Tumor growth is related to the proportion of mitotic activity and apoptotic and/or necroptotic or necrotic cell proportion (H&E, original magnification ×40)

are recognized by neighbor cells and macrophages, by which they are phagocytosed and degraded.

Apoptosis may be activated by intrinsic pathway by DNA damage, hypoxia, and decrease in hormonal stimuli or by extrinsic pathway by the binding of the death signals (e.g., tumor necrosis factor alpha) to death receptors. During carcinogenesis, the regulatory mechanisms of apoptosis are also disturbed resulting in the decrease of apoptosis. Tumor growth is not only related to increased proliferation but also decreased apoptosis.

The two pathways, extrinsic and intrinsic, that are important in apoptotic switch may both be effected in cells with malignant transformation; multiple steps of apoptosis may be the following:

- p53 mutations are frequent in carcinomas, and loss of p53 function results in functional reduction of pro-apoptotic factors, like BAX.
- Upregulation of antiapoptotic factors BCL-2, BCL-X2, and MCL-1 keeps cytochrome c in the mitochondria.
- Loss of apoptotic peptidase activating factor.
- Upregulators of the inhibitors of apoptosis like X-linked inhibitor of apoptosis protein (XIAP) which inhibits the activation of caspases by binding to them. These factors are important in both inhibition of intrinsic and extrinsic pathways, and their expressions are induced with oncogenes, like Ras.
- Inactivation of death-induced signaling complex; Fas associated via death domain (FADD) is important in extrinsic apoptotic pathway.
- CD95, a death receptor and a member of the subgroup of tumor necrosis factor superfamily, which is important in extrinsic apoptotic pathway by association of FADD and proforms of caspases 8 and 10, is reduced.

All of these changes contribute to the decline of apoptosis in carcinomas. Decrease in apoptosis or resistance to stimuli that is targeted for the induction of apoptosis is important for strategies in patient treatment as well as survival (Goldar et al. 2015, Su et al. 2015; Kumar V et al. 2015).

Anoikis

Anoikis means homelessness. Under normal conditions, loss of cell adhesion induces apoptosis. Integrins function as growth factor receptors, and loss of the intercellular adhesion stimuli results in cell death, and this is named as anoikis. It is a mechanism that prevents survival of the cells that have lost their adhesions and somehow disseminated in blood flow; again this is a mechanism in normal life, first observed in endothelial and epithelial cells. This mechanism avoids distant colonization of cells.

Tumor cells are also prone to anoikis, if they don't have mechanisms that save them from this basic mechanism. Anchorage-independent survival, escape from anoikis, may be with multiple mechanisms in tumor cells, like changes in integrin expressions, activation of many survival signals related to sustained autocrine loops, activation of the oncogenes, and overexpression of the growth factors. Mutations or upregulation of the integrins and growth factor receptor signaling may prevent anoikis. While the disseminated tumor cells rest in the tumor niche, the extracellular matrix may contribute to the survival or anoikis resistance, by modulating EMT and metabolic changes (Gilmore 2005; Paoli et al. 2013).

Necroptosis

Necrosis was considered to be an unregulated process; however, recent evidence highlights a multistep mechanism which may be activated by tumor necrosis factor supergene family, T cells, interferon, Toll-like receptors, as well as different types of cellular stresses including chemotherapeutics. This particular process is named as programmed cell necrosis or *necroptosis*. Like apoptosis, necroptosis is activated by the death receptor tumor necrosis factor receptor superfamily as well as other mechanisms including that of Fas and viral DNA or RNA, but it is not related to the activation of caspases. Necroptosis should be differentiated from necrosis which is related to physical trauma like heat, ischemia, and pathogens. Like apoptosis, necroptosis is also a basic mechanism in development. Receptor-interacting protein kinase (RIP) 1 and 3 are important in the formation of "necrosome," the characteristic structure of this process. RIP1 is also important in the induction of inflammation, particularly if caspase 8 activity is absent.

If stressful conditions like ATP depletion, increased reactive oxygen species, hypoxia, or DNA damage are mild, they may induce autophagy, but if these are severe, they may induce apoptosis, or if they are more severe, then necroptosis may be triggered. Same stimuli may induce either apoptosis or necroptosis in different conditions, like different pHs.

Dysregulation of necroptosis machinery seems to be a feature of carcinomas. RIP1 gene polymorphism may be associated with some types of malignancies. Necroptosis is an antimetastatic mechanism like apoptosis (Zhou and Yuan 2014; Su et al. 2015).

Proteases: Degradation of the Extratumoral Spaces

Serine proteases, matrix metalloproteinases (MMPs), and their tissue inhibitors (TIMPs) act by balancing their activities during normal cellular functions. During tumor progression, MMPs are important in the degradation of the basement membrane increasing sequentially from preneoplastic lesions to carcinoma in situ and invasive tumor (Sarioğlu et al. 2001). Increased MMP expressions were found to be poor prognostic factors in different types of carcinomas (Sis et al. 2004, Cavdar et al. 2011). Stromal cells also contribute to the expression of these proteases, helping to increase the invasive and metastatic phenotype.

Epithelial-Mesenchymal Transition

Epithelial-mesenchymal transition (EMT) is a complex but basic mechanism at different phases in life including embryogenesis and development. It is also important in pathological conditions like in wound healing and fibrosis (Kalluri and Weinberg 2009, Tiwari N et al. 2012, Rybinski et al. 2014). EMT is the morphological and functional alteration of many aspects of a cell. The epithelial cells that line all the inner and outer surfaces of the body are attached to each other and the basement membrane. The basement membrane supports the epithelial cells and also forms a barrier that does not allow the passage of the epithelial cells to the subepithelial, submucosal, or subepidermal region. Epithelial cells grow to the opposite direction of the basement membrane, forming basal-apical polarity. The histopathologists name the crossing of the basement membrane by epithelial cells as "invasion" in malignant transformation, and this is one of the hallmarks of malignancy (Fig. 1.5); however, it is not a mutually exclusive phenomenon for the malignant cells; other cells can also perform this as a part of development and homeostasis (Hay 1995, Kalluri and Weinberg 2009).

During EMT the expression of intermediate filament cytokeratin, reflecting epithelial differentiation, decreases as well as E-cadherin which is important in intercellular junctions and laminin which is a component of the basement membrane along with a set of molecules, while another group of markers that are associated with mesenchymal differentiation increases including vimentin. Many regulators take part during this transition, like Snail, a transcription factor important in the regulation of cadherins, inducing the repression of the expression of E-cadherin. A set of markers associated with epithelial and mesenchymal cells are listed in Table 1.1. The mesenchymal phenotype allows the epithelial cells to have many new abilities including invasiveness, elevated resistance to apoptosis, and greatly increased production of ECM components, and these features give the cell the capacity of migration. The latter features all remind us of the malignant transformation; in order to differentiate these processes under different conditions, a three-tiered classification is proposed (Kalluri and Weinberg 2009):

Type I: EMT in embryogenesis. Embryogenesis is a stage of life enriched with EMT. Even implantation during embryogenesis requires EMT. Wnt pathway is important at this stage. As an example, the melanocytes, which are derived from epithelial cells from the neuroectoderm, give rise to migratory neural crest cells; from there, during migration to the skin, EMT is the basic mechanism. The transition is transient and is not associated with fibrosis.

Type II: EMT in regeneration and fibrosis. Phenotypical changes like EMT are observed during the development of fibrosis. During the development of fibrosis, like in renal diseases, excessive alpha-smooth muscle actin expression is expected. Due to this, the process was named as epithelial myofibroblastic transformation. These mechanisms also operate during the fibrosing processes in the liver, lung, and intestine (Kirimca et al. 2001, Kalluri and Weinberg 2009). This

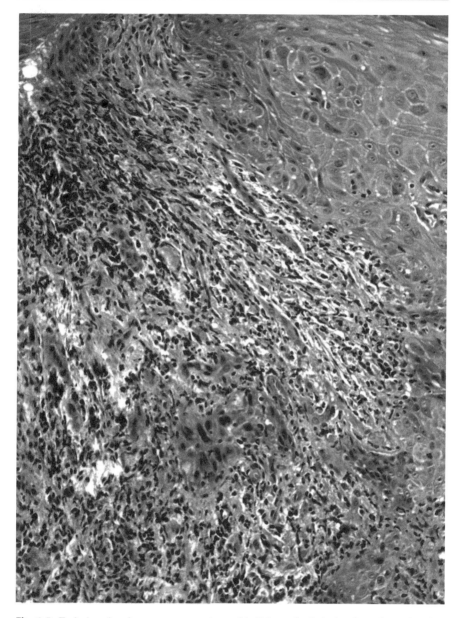

Fig. 1.5 Early invasion from a squamous intraepithelial neoplastic lesion from the oral cavity. There is inflammatory reaction and loss of the integrity of the basement membrane (H&E, original magnification ×20)

Table 1.1 The markers that are related to epithelial or mesenchymal phenotype during epithelial to mesenchymal transition (Banyard and Bielenberg 2015, Tiwari N et al. 2012)

	Epithelial	Mesenchymal
Markers	Cytokeratins, epithelial membrane antigen, E-cadherin, P-cadherin, ZO-1, EpCAM, occludin, claudins 3,4,7, laminin 1, desmoplakin, entactin, desmocollin 2,3, syndecan 1, γ-catenin, integrin β4, miR-200	Vimentin, α-smooth muscle actin, N-cadherin, nuclear β-catenin, fibronectin, MMP2,3,9, TCFC4, LEF-1, SOX1, SIX1, Snail (SNAI1), Slug (SNAI2), twist, FSP1/S100A4, goosecoid, FOXC2, ZEB1, integrins α5β1,αvβ6, GATA 3, miR-21

mechanism is associated with tissue injury and inflammation; EMT seems to continue as long as the inducing factor persists and production of extensive amounts of collagen rich stroma is a typical feature (Rybinski et al. 2014).

Type III: This type of EMT is the one associated with neoplasia. The invasion through the basement membrane and metastasis are associated with EMT. This transition is induced by the genomic changes acquired during the neoplastic transformation (Kalluri and Weinberg 2009). The neoplastic cells also acquire stem cell-like properties. However, it must be kept in mind that the cells which are not at the same EMT stage are not the same with each other. Although loss of cytokeratins and increase in vimentin are common features, other markers may be expressed at different levels reflecting different degrees of EMT (Banyard and Bielenberg 2015).

EMT Regulation

The regulation of EMT is related to many factors that may be accepted in three groups, inducers, regulators, and effectors:

Inducers

- Autocrine growth factors secreted by the neoplastic cells, EGF, HGF, FGF, and TGFβ, bind to respective receptor tyrosine kinases to induce EMT and to elicit an invasive and migratory state.
- The hypoxic tumor center induced angiogenic mediators that induce EMT, including VEGF, IGF, TGFβ, HGF, FGF, Wnt, and Notch.
- Inflammation induced by the tumor brings cytokines (TNFα, IFNγ, IL6, and IL1β) that induce the expression of transcription factors such as Snail and zinc finger E-box-binding homeobox (ZEB), which are important in EMT and metastasis (Banyard and Bielenberg 2015, Tiwari N et al. 2012).

Regulators

- The TF families (zinc finger proteins Snail and Slug), zinc finger and homeodomain proteins (ZEB1 and ZEB2), and Twist (basic helix-loop-helix proteins E12, E47, Twist1 Twist2, and Id) are transcription factors that repress transcription of E-cadherin.
- In TGFβ-driven EMT which is mostly seen in type II EMT, transcription factors such as SMAD and BMP are important in opposite ways.
- HIF1α associated with hypoxia is an important EMT inducer.
- GATA, SOX, and forkhead box (FOX) proteins seem to play a role in EMT.
- microRNAs function by gene silencing in EMT (Banyard and Bielenberg 2015).

Effectors

- Cell junction changes:
  - Changes in tight, gap, adherens junctions, desmosomes, as well as hemidesmosomes
  - Cadherin switches, E-cadherin to N-cadherin
  - Catenin, claudin, desmocollin, and JAM changes
- Cell skeleton changes of intermediate filaments: shift from cytokeratin to vimentin resulting in changes in cellular morphology, such as becoming spindle shaped.
- Upregulation of collagenases (MMP2, MMP9, MMP13) for destruction of the extracellular matrix.
- Expression of factors preventing anoikis (apoptosis of epithelial cells which have lost intercellular connections with other epithelial cells): this is regulated including PI3K/AKT, NF-κB, Wnt/β-catenin, and p53/p63 pathways.
- Drug resistance and escaping from the immune mechanisms of the host are also related to EMT (Banyard and Bielenberg 2015, Morgillo et al. 2016).

However, EMT does not seem to be a prerequisite for tumor metastasis as once thought, as what the studies on CTCs have shown on the expression of epithelial markers. Then it was suggested that "partial EMT" may also be a feature associated with metastatic phenotype (Alix-Panabières et al. 2017).

Mesenchymal-Epithelial Transition

EMT is reversible; that's why it is named as transition but not transformation. The information about EMT is much more than MET. There is convincing evidence about EMT during the process of invasion and entry to the blood vessels; however, the metastatic tumor clusters do not have EMT properties. Most of the evidence about MET is related to in vitro experiments and experimental models (Banyard and Bielenberg 2015). It is suggested that, at the stage of EMT, tumor cells cannot form metastatic colonies; they have to transit to the epithelial stage with MET (Alix-Panabières et al. 2017).

EMT, Stem Cells, and Tumor-Initiating Cells

Cancer tissue is made up of a mixture of cells creating an ecosystem including endothelial, stromal, and inflammatory cells as well as the carcinoma cells. The malignant cells are also heterogeneous, and this seems to be related to genetic and epigenetic events and tumor microenvironment. All tumor cells cannot initiate a metastatic population or a xenograft tumor.

Tumor stem cells share many features with the stem cells of the normal tissues. Stemness is a collective term for integrated function of molecular programs that lead and maintain stem cell features. Each tumor has different proportions of intra-tumoral cells that may initiate a new tumor at a distant site, and these are named as tumor-initiating cells (TIC). TIC are different from stem cells. Stemness and therapy resistance were shown to be associated in different types of tumors, like colon and breast carcinomas, as well as increased proliferation, metastasizing, and self-renewal capacity (Clevers 2011, Kreso and Dick 2014).

Stem cells share some features with tumor cells with EMT. They are both induced by TNFβ, and they are resistant to chemotherapy. Like the gradient of EMT, there may be a gradient of stemness.

It takes about 10 days, for a cell to acquire all features of EMT at in vitro models (Tiwari et al. 2012). It seems EMT is a mechanism of particular importance in tumor metastasis and MET also seems to be required for metastasis; however, these do not have to be the only mechanisms for metastasis.

Cell Adhesion

Cellular adhesion and the molecules that mediate these processes, cellular adhesion molecules (CAM), are important in both physiological processes and many steps during carcinogenesis, invasion, and metastasis. Cellular adhesion may be in two forms cell-cell (homophilic) and cell-matrix (heterophilic). The adhesion molecules may be grouped as follows:

- Cadherins: Molecules expressed in cells with some specific organ or cell-type distributions like epithelial, neural, placental, etc. However each molecule may be expressed at different concentrations in many cells. They bind to intracellular actin by β-catenin.
- Integrins: Molecules expressed extensively at the extracellular matrix, connecting extracellular components like collagen, fibronectin, etc. Although these molecules are expressed at the extracellular area, they have effects on differentiation, apoptosis, and survival. Collagen and fibrin induce the change of integrins to high-affinity state, and this is important in platelet aggregation.

- Immunoglobulin superfamily: This is a rather large family, and the immuno-globulins are the first subgroup. Cellular adhesion molecules include neural cell adhesion molecules (NCAM), intercellular adhesion molecule (ICAM), and CD2 subset (CD48, CD58, CD50, CD229, CD244).
- Addressins (lymphocyte homing receptor): GLYCAM-1 and CD34 are in this group.
- Selectins: These heterophilic adhesion molecules may be endothelial (E-selectin), platelet related (P-selectin), and leucocyte related (L-selectin). They bind to fucosylated carbohydrates.

Intercellular and basement membrane adhesion molecules are important in the polarized structure of the epithelium. Intercellular adhesion molecule E-cadherin is very important in EMT as well as MET. Loss of E-cadherin may happen with many mechanisms including inactivating mutations of either deletion or loss as well as promoter hypermethylation. Considering the EMT and MET even during embryo-genesis, we may think of a switch of the expression of E-cadherin. There is a recip-rocal expression of N-cadherin with E-cadherin; it is thought that their expressions are related. N-cadherin induces the expression of N-cadherin by stromal cells and is an inducer of malignant cell invasion and diapedesis.

β-catenin is tied to the cytoplasmic tail of E-cadherin. The activation of Wnt signaling pathway results in the placement in the nucleus, and there, it induces cell proliferation through c-myc and cyclin D1, and mutant β-catenin may induce EMT through the expression of molecules like Snail and Slug.

The invasion of the tumor cells destroying the basement membrane, with loss of intercellular adhesion, is followed by the encounter with the stroma, and still tumor cells use adhesion molecules.

If the intravascular tumor cells are traveling as clusters (still expressing E-cadherin for intercellular adhesion), they may be more resistant to pressure and may escape from natural killer T cells. The different surface adhesion molecules, some of which are named as tumor antigens, are expressed by the tumor cells like carcinoembryonic antigen, CD44, and podocalyxin, and these are the sites associ-ated with P-selectin and integrin adhesion molecular binding, resulting in platelet and leukocyte aggregation on tumor cells allowing escape of the circulating tumor cell clusters from the immune surveillance. The endothelial cells express P- and E-selectins in case they are activated, and these receptors capture tumor cells or clusters. Vascular endothelial cadherin (VE-cadherin) and the platelet-endothelial cell adhesion molecule-l (PECAM- l) are involved in endothelial cell adhesion and in the formation of inter-endothelial junctions, related to lumen formation and per-meability (Balzer and Konstantopoulos 2012, Singh et al. 2015).

Different roles of tumor-related molecules are being uncovered; for example, CD44 was evaluated as a prognostic marker as an adhesion molecule previously in different types of carcinomas; however, it is now thought of as a marker of stemness (Sökmen et al. 2001a, b; Yan et al. 2015).

Tumor-Stroma Interactions

Tumor microenvironment includes cancer-associated fibroblasts (CAFs), inflammatory cells, endothelial cells, and mesenchymal stem cells as well as extracellular matrix components, all of which are important in tumor progression (Fig. 1.6). CAFs are suggested to be derived from endothelial, epithelial, and smooth muscle cells and have strong contractile properties. These cells are said to be educated by the tumor cells in order to act in a fashion that is suitable for tumor growth.

CAFs cleave ECM components; secrete matrix metalloproteinases (MMPs) that degrade the extracellular matrix, as well as TGF-β and HGF inducing EMT in cancer cells; and present exosomes to cancer cells promoting invasive phenotype. Actin-rich membrane protrusions of the tumor cells are named as invadopodia; these localize MMP activity increasing invasive potential. CAFs contribute to matrix stiffening through actomyosin contractility and ECM secretion, and this property of the matrix enhances integrin-mediated mechanotransduction (Yamaguchi and Sakai 2015). Co-cultures of fibroblasts and squamous cell carcinoma cells

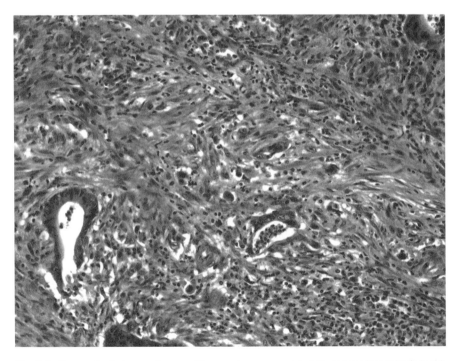

Fig. 1.6 Desmoplastic tumor stroma with many tumor-associated fibroblasts intermingled with malignant isolated tumor cells and glands from a rectal adenocarcinoma case (H&E, original magnification ×40)

showed the co-invasion of both cells and, even more, the leading cells were the fibroblasts (Gaggioli et al. 2007). Furthermore, stromal cells were also found to express CD44 under stringent conditions like hypoxia leading to the stemness of both CAFs and tumor cells (Kinugasa et al. 2014).

Tumor-stroma ratio or increased desmoplasia was found to be a poor prognostic factor in different types of tumors, colorectal carcinomas in particular (Sis B 2005; West et al. 2010); however, there are controversial results in different types of carcinomas (Unlu et al. 2013, Gurel et al. 2016). Lymphoid tumors and Hodgkin's lymphoma in particular are also associated with fibrotic stromal response (Tataroglu et al. 2007).

Escape from Immune Surveillance

Congenital and acquired immune deficiency states are associated with increased risk of malignant tumor progression and poor prognosis (Mapara and Sykes 2004).

Immune system may function in different pathways at different stages of tumor progression. These may be summarized at three phases:

- Elimination: Innate and adaptive immune systems recognize malignant cells and eliminate them before any type of clinical manifestations. Tumor-associated antigens and tumor-specific antigens are important for the recognition. Tumor-infiltrating lymphocytes (TILs) are associated with increased mutations and better survival. Tumor regression with clonal expansion of T cells in malignant melanomas suggests the importance of the immune system.
- Equilibrium: The immune system may suppress the tumor growth, and the tumor stays in dormancy.
- Escape: Tumor cells use mechanisms for escaping immune system and thus can grow and metastasize. Reduced immune recognition, resistance to attacks of the immune system, and immune suppressive tumor microenvironment may contribute to "escape" of the tumor cells. Selection of the tumor cells with least immunogenicity and ones that suppress the immune system results in proliferation of clones with increased capacity to escape. Tumor regulatory T cells (Tregs) suppress autoimmunity under physiological conditions, and these may contribute to immune suppression during tumor progression. Necrotic tissue fragments activate Tregs, and these cells are capable of suppressing T cells and B cells including cytotoxic T cells. Tumor-secreted factors induce the entrained neutrophils (TENs), and these are also important in prevention of metastasis, especially in early stages (Granot et al. 2011).

Stimulation of the immune system has always attracted the attention of oncologists. Immunotherapy by vaccines and immune checkpoint inhibitors, targeting cytotoxic T-lymphocyte antigen 4 (CTLA-4), programmed death-1 (PD-1), and programmed death-ligand (PDL), seems to have important contributions to the treatment of patients with positivity of these markers (Muenst et al. 2016; Snyder et al. 2014, Topalian et al. 2012, Sgambato et al. 2016).

Metastasis

The title of this section is "Metastasis"; however, many features were discussed in the previous pages. It is hard to describe the structure, behavior, and function of the carcinoma cells without referring to the features of the process of metastasis.

Fortunately not all cancer cells are capable of starting metastatic colonies. The first steps in carcinoma progression, invasion, and angiogenesis are also important for metastasis.

The sequential and interconnected events during metastasis start with detachment followed by migration and invasion; however, these are basically features of invasion. Lymphatic and vascular invasion and traveling are the frequently listed pathways, but generally others like perineural invasion, perivascular invasion, pagetoid spread, and seeding are neglected (Sarioglu et al. 2016). In the next chapter, the latter three mechanisms will be discussed. If we consider only the lymphatic and blood vessel metastasis, a few additional points should be discussed in addition to the information in the previous pages.

The tumor cells should attach to the vessels and overcome anoikis and immune surveillance in order to travel by lymphatics and/or blood vessels, attach to the vessel walls, penetrate to the extravascular space, and start a new growth.

Tumor Migration

During migration, different types of movements were described:

- *Single-cell migration*: Cells that have undergone EMT adhere to the ECM with integrins, expressing proteases, and contraction of the intracytoplasmic actin and myosin filaments allows the movement of the cell.
- *Collective cell migration*: Collective cell migration is an alternative mechanism that should be kept in mind. Cells with less predominant EMT may use amoeboid movement during migration. This is a feature that may be seen in head and neck squamous cell carcinomas; it was suggested that podoplanin expression by tumor cell clusters growing like fingers induced filopodia formation and cell migration; also podoplanin was suggested to have a similar function in breast carcinomas (Diepenbruck and Christofori 2016, Banyard and Bielenberg 2015). Observation of monoclonal but heterogeneous metastatic and micrometastatic foci argues against metastasis by single cells and highlights instead the role of collective cell migration in metastasis. However, at least at the leading edges, they have some degree of EMT features (Lambert et al. 2017).

Single-tumor-cell metastasis is a favored mechanism coined with EMT, and passing of the tumor cell clusters through the capillary walls was a debatable issue; however, recently it has been shown that extravasation of clusters up to 20 cells is possible, in experimental models with microfluidic devices mimicking capillaries (Au et al. 2016).

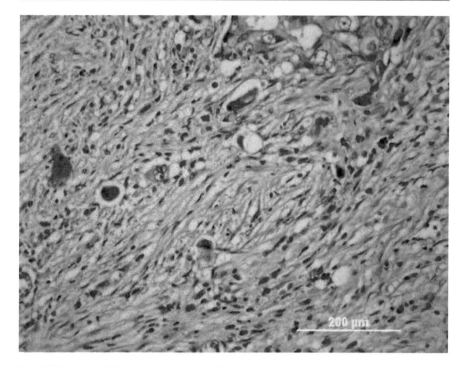

Fig. 1.7 Tumor budding: groups of 1–5 dedifferentiated tumor cells surrounded by desmoplastic stroma

Tumor budding is a morphological tumor feature associated with poor progno-sis in different types of carcinomas (Sarioglu et al. 2010). There are controversies about the methods of assessment of budding, but the most favored of them is as follows: Tumor buds are accepted as 1–5 dedifferentiated tumor cells surrounded by desmoplastic stroma, discontinuous with the main tumor mass. It was shown in three-dimensional reconstructions that fingerlike projections of the tumors infil-trate the invasive tumor front and at the end these buds detach from the main tumor mass (Fig. 1.7). The cells have lower ki-67 index and increased p16, cyclin-D1, β-catenin, and CD133 expressions compared with the main tumor, consistent with the concepts of "grow or go" (proliferative arrest of the cells during metastasis) and achieving stem cell features during invasion and metastasis. These features of the budding cells seem to be like a cell with partial EMT and stem cell features (Grigore et al. 2016).

Circulating Tumor Cells

Circulating tumor cells (CTCs) are found to have many features of a cell with EMT, both in experimental studies and breast carcinoma patients (Yu et al. 2013). CTCs provide valuable information in many aspects. Their half-life in blood is thought to be 1–2.4 h, and one of the mechanisms for their loss is extravasation. Many factors are important to their fate:

- The pressure in blood vessels is an important stress factor.
- The immune system's performance is important in CTC evasion. T cells are important in defense against the tumors; if the CTCs express PD-L1, they bind to the PD receptors in T cells, inhibiting T-cell proliferation and cytokine production (Alix-Panabières et al. 2017).
- Platelets may cover the CTCs and they are thought to induce a more EMT phenotype. This process also helps the tumor cells to hide from immune system. The coverage with platelets may affect the endothelial cells to retract and allow transendothelial migration (Lambert et al. 2017).

Although the research in CTCs is promising, the characteristics of the tumor cells at different stages of EMT or MET make the detection and separation of the tumor cells difficult. However different technologies are being employed for this purpose (Alix-Panabières et al. 2017). DNA isolation from CTCs obtained by liquid biopsies, "blood samples," may allow detection of ongoing mutations in tumoral mass; however, its value in clinical practice is not settled yet (Sholl et al. 2016).

Autophagy may inhibit metastasis at the early carcinogenesis by saving the cells from necrosis, inflammation, and oncogene-induced senescence. On the other hand, it supports the detachment of the cancer cells from ECM and colonization at other sites and induces dormancy under unfavorable conditions.

Increasing the fitness of the tumor cells under stressful conditions, autophagy saves the cells from both apoptosis and necroptosis as well as immune cell infiltration (Su et al. 2015; Lambert et al. 2017).

Metastasis Suppressor Genes

Metastasis suppressor genes are the genes that do not influence tumor growth but are important in metastasis. Comparative analysis of the loss of heterozygosity (LOH) at tumors at different stages followed by microcell-mediated chromosomal transfer as well as subtractive hybridization, differential display, and comparative genomic hybridization methods was applied during the identification of genes with tumor suppressor properties. The metastasis suppressor genes may be grouped into three:

- Transcriptional regulators [e.g., breast cancer metastasis suppressor-1 (BCMS-1)]
- Posttranscriptional regulators [e.g., metastasis-related miRNAs (metastamiR), tissue inhibitor of matrix metalloproteinases (TIMPs)]
- Regulators of cellular communication [e.g., CD44, E-cadherin, KAI-1, deleted in colorectal cancer-1 (DCC-1), Nm23]

Nm23 is the first identified metastasis suppressor gene; however, still the mechanism, probably prevention of MAPK pathway, is important. The expression of the metastasis suppressor genes in carcinomas is associated with better prognosis, and they have suppressor effects on tumor through angiogenesis, EMT, transport, migration, motility, intravasation, as well as colonization. Mutation of these genes is rare. Their expression is frequently downregulated (Hurst and Welch 2011).

Exosomes in Cancer Metastasis

The discoveries related to "exosomes," small vesicles transporting different types of molecules in the cell, brought the Nobel Prize in 2013 to three scientists: James Rothman, Randy Schekman, and Thomas Sudhof. Their functions are remarkable at a cell at homeostasis, as they transport the required things at the right time to the right place, as a tiny 30–100 nm envelope, carried by a careful postman, and might better be named as "endosomes" if they have intracellular function. They may provide directional transport from the basement of the cell to the lumen in a polarized cell as well as carrying waste products to lysosomes. The exosomes may carry many different things in autocrine, paracrine, and endocrine fashion. If they arise from malignant cells, they may contain many things like oncogene-coded RNAs and proteins, growth factors, and different types of miRNAs. It is thought that if they act in an extracellular position in case of neoplasia, they may carry the stuff to possible sites of metastasis and induce a niche formation that could welcome the metastatic population (Banyard and Bielenberg 2015).

Invasion of the Vessels

Lymphatic vessels are different from the blood vessels. At the distal end, they do not have pericytes or basement membranes. Increased interstitial pressure induces the opening of the "button junctions." The lack of both layers surrounding the lymphatics and button junctions allows much more easier access of the tumor cells to the lymphatic tumor compared with an arterial structure (Baluk et al. 2007). Arterioles are surrounded by basement membranes and pericytes, and these structures get thicker and stronger at the larger arterial vessels. In order to invade these vascular structures, tumor cells must have strong degrading capacity (Figs. 1.8, 1.9, and 1.10). It is easier for the tumor cells to invade the leaky, newly formed vessels, the products of angiogenesis. During the tumor growth, at some point, some parts of the tumor get hypoxic, and hypoxic tumor center cells express angiogenic and lymphangiogenic factors. The peritumoral lymphatics were found to have 10–50 times larger diameters than their normal tissue counterparts; this may be due to pressure differences caused by the tumor mass or the growth factors secreted by the tumor cells. The lymphatic system provides a better environment for the tumor cells, as the lymphatic endothelial cells secrete chemotactic agents and the low pressure and low flow rate are better for the survival of the tumor cells compared with the blood vessels (Zwaans and Bielenberg 2007).

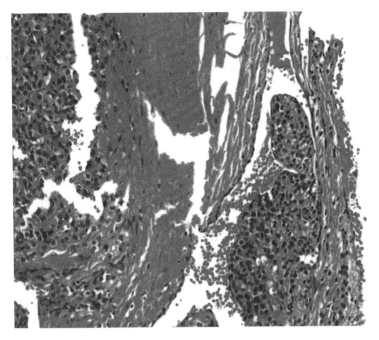

Fig. 1.8 Vascular invasion, note the attachment of the huge metastatic colony to the endothelium (H&E, original magnification ×20)

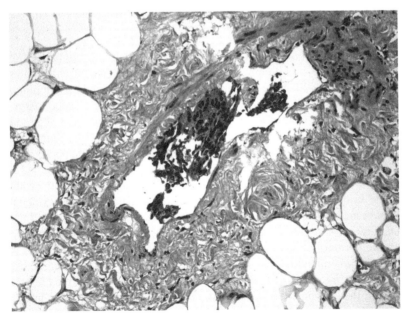

Fig. 1.9 Vascular invasion, note the attachment of the huge metastatic colony to the endothelium at multiple points (H&E, original magnification ×20)

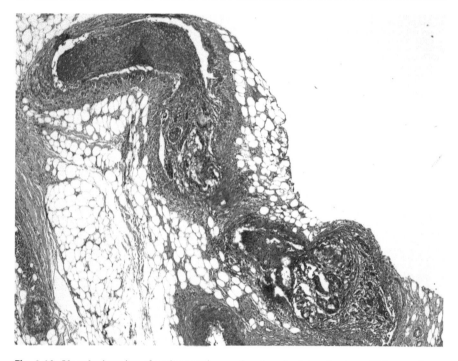

Fig. 1.10 Vascular invasion of a adenocarcinoma, forming glandular structures. This case shows that without epithelial-mesenchymal transition, vascular invasion and migration may take place. The intravascular mass is covered with fibrin trombi (H&E, original magnification ×10)

Lymphatic metastasis is the first metastatic site of the epithelial tumors. Finding tumor cells in a lymphatic does not mean metastasis; it only shows that some of the tumor cells have the capacity of separation from the main tumor and enter the lymphatic (Figs. 1.11, 1.12, and 1.13). Even seeing isolated tumor cells at a lymph node is not sufficient for a diagnosis of metastasis as they may be bypassers. If the tumor cells form a population of 0.2–2.00 mm diameter, then this is named as micrometastasis, and this does not correlate with poor prognosis. The lymph node (or nodes), where the tumor's lymphatic drains, is named as the "sentinel lymph node." If this node is negative, the lymph nodes at the route are expected to be tumor-free. This concept is used in patient treatment mainly in malignant melanoma and breast carcinomas, and there are applications for other organ tumors (Chen et al. 2006). Antilymphangiogenic therapies that do not affect the normal lymphatics are being targeted toward the prevention of tumor metastasis. It is noted that the cells invading lymphatics show decreased expression of vimentin compared to the cells at the invasive borders of the tumors. It is suggested that lymphatic invasion may be caused by cells that have not undergone EMT, but the cells that have undergone EMT may also cause lymphatic invasion; however, it seems it is easier for metastatic colonies of cells to grow without EMT (Banyard and Bielenberg 2015).

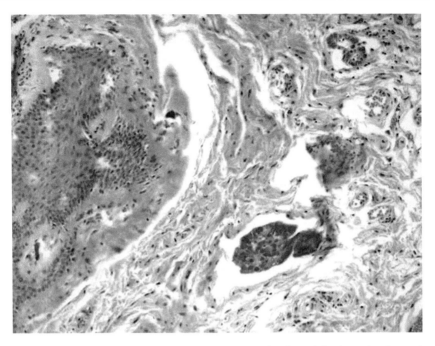

Fig. 1.11 Lymphatic invasion at the distal surgical margin of an abdominoperineal resection patient (H&E, original magnification ×20)

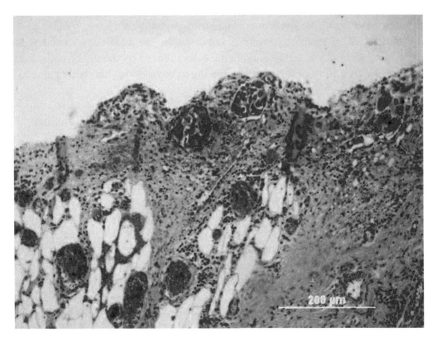

Fig. 1.12 Lymphatic invasion at the submesothelial region of a colectomy specimen (H&E, original magnification ×20)

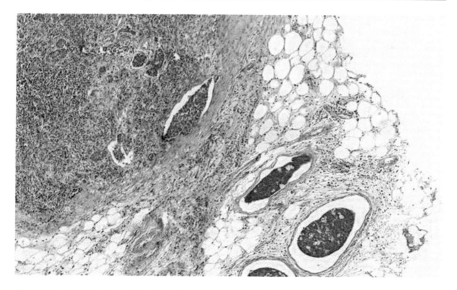

Fig. 1.13 Multiple lymphatic invasion at a neuroendocrine carcinoma patient (H&E, original magnification ×10)

Extravasation

Expressions of multiple mediators, including angiopoietinlike-4, VEGF, MMPs, ADAM12, CCL2, platelets covering tumor cells, metastasis-associated macrophages, and necroptosis of the endothelial cells induced by the tumor cells, lead to increased permeability of the vessels allowing extravasation (Lambert et al. 2017).

Metastatic Colonization, Tumor Dormancy, and Reactivation

Synchronous and metachronous metastasis depend upon different mechanisms, at least partially. It may be easier to understand synchronous growth, but what stops the tumor metastasis for many years, sometimes decades, like in same patients with malignant melanoma and breast or prostatic carcinoma, and what starts the tumor cell growth after such long periods are more complex questions (Fig. 1.14). There is experimental evidence that tumor cells may be found in the circulation, even if the neoplasia is at a noninvasive stage, and it is suggested that early dissemination and dormancy are features of many types of carcinomas. Primary tumor dormancy may be related to oncogene-induced senescence, immune surveillance, and/or waiting for the angiogenic switch. As mentioned above, the cells stop proliferative activity during the process of metastasis, and this is named as proliferative quiescence. Turning back to proliferative phase seems to be delayed at isolated tumor cells.

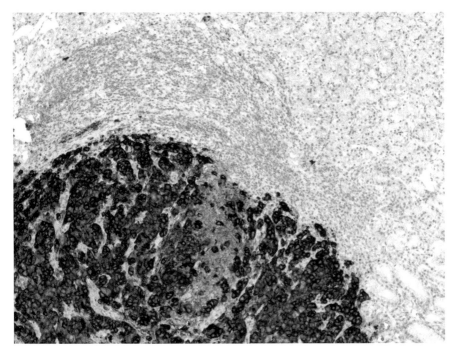

Fig. 1.14 Metachronous metastasis at unexpected sites is a feature of malignant melanoma. This patient had a skin malignant melanoma diagnosis 9 years ago. During the endoscopy many submucosal small nodules were observed and biopsied. Note the submucosal atypical cells with strong HMB-45 expression. The cells that were carried to this site nearly a decade ago lived in dormancy at the tumor niche, to wake up to produce these neoplastic mass lesions (IHC, HMB-45, original magnification ×20)

Additionally the new tumor microenvironment is distinctly different from the primary location (Figure metastasis melanoma). If these cells start proliferation to produce micrometastatic nodules, the immune system may cause elimination or equilibrium of the tumor cells, as brakes to metastatic tumor growth. The hormonal antagonists may prevent tumor growth as in breast and prostatic carcinomas; hormonal deprivation may be one of the reasons of tumor dormancy (Gao et al. 2012; Giancotti 2013).

The place where the dormant cells reside is named as "tumor niche," the place that supports the survival, dormancy, and stem-like features. In many cases, the niche is at the perivascular region which may be under the influence of thrombospondin-1 secreted by the endothelial cells (Lambert et al. 2017).

The cells that will start a new colony at a distant site should have or acquire the properties of stem cells or tumor-initiating cells, the cells that are resistant to chemotherapy. Stromal inhibitory factors like BMP and the lack of the activating factors like Wnt and Notch seem to be important in dormancy. The reciprocal expression may lead to activation (Gao et al. 2012; Giancotti 2013).

Last Words

There is a wide accumulation of information on cells, tissues, and organisms during physiological conditions and neoplastic conditions. It was not possible to refer to all the excellent studies that enlightened us during the scientific fight against cancer. This is an incomplete wall that is being built by many scientists, adding blocks, that is rising against cancer. A brief summary of the events is presented in Fig. 1.15.

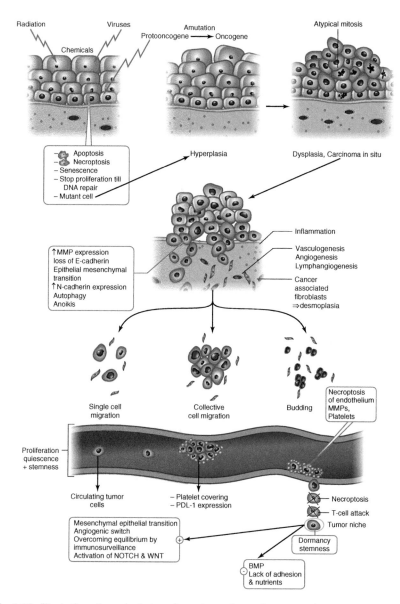

Fig. 1.15 Illustration of neoplastic transformation and vascular metastasis

References

Alix-Panabières C, Mader S, Pantel K. Epithelial-mesenchymal plasticity in circulating tumor cells. J Mol Med (Berl). 2017;95(2):133–42. https://doi.org/10.1007/s00109-016-1500-6. Review. PubMed PMID: 28013389.

Au SH, Storey BD, Moore JC, Tang Q, Chen YL, Javaid S, Sarioglu AF, Sullivan R, Madden MW, O'Keefe R, Haber DA, Maheswaran S, Langenau DM, Stott SL, Toner M. Clusters of circulating tumor cells traverse capillary-sized vessels. Proc Natl Acad Sci U S A. 2016;113(18):4947–52. https://doi.org/10.1073/pnas.1524448113. PubMed PMID: 27091969; PubMed Central PMCID: PMC4983862.

Baluk P, Fuxe J, Hashizume H, Romano T, Lashnits E, Butz S, Vestweber D, Corada M, Molendini C, Dejana E, McDonald DM. Functionally specialized junctions between endothelial cells of lymphatic vessels. J Exp Med. 2007;204(10):2349–62. PubMed PMID: 17846148; PubMed Central PMCID: PMC2118470.

Balzer EM, Konstantopoulos K. Intercellular adhesion: mechanisms for growth and metastasis of epithelial cancers. Wiley Interdiscip Rev Syst Biol Med. 2012;4(2):171–81. https://doi.org/10.1002/wsbm.160. Review. PubMed PMID: 21913338; PubMed Central PMCID: PMC4476647.

Banyard J, Bielenberg DR. The role of EMT and MET in cancer dissemination. Connect Tissue Res. 2015;56(5):403–13. https://doi.org/10.3109/03008207.2015.1060970. Review. PubMed PMID: 26291767; PubMed Central PMCID: PMC4780319.

Bridgeman VL, Vermeulen PB, Foo S, Bilecz A, Daley F, Kostaras E, Nathan MR, Wan E, Frentzas S, Schweiger T, Hegedus B, Hoetzenecker K, Renyi-Vamos F, Kuczynski EA, Vasudev NS, Larkin J, Gore M, Dvorak HF, Paku S, Kerbel RS, Dome B, Reynolds AR. Vessel co-option is common in human lung metastases and mediates resistance to anti-angiogenic therapy in preclinical lung metastasis models. J Pathol. 2017;241(3):362–74. https://doi.org/10.1002/path.4845. PubMed PMID: 27859259.

Cavdar Z, Canda AE, Terzi C, Sarioglu S, Fuzun M, Oktay G. Role of gelatinases (matrix metalloproteinases 2 and 9), vascular endothelial growth factor and endostatin on clinicopathological behaviour of rectal cancer. Color Dis. 2011;13(2):154–60. https://doi.org/10.1111/j.1463-1318.2009.02105.x. PubMed PMID: 19888958.

Chen SL, Iddings DM, Scheri RP, Bilchik AJ. Lymphatic mapping and sentinel node analysis: current concepts and applications. CA Cancer J Clin. 2006;56(5):292–309. Quiz 316–7. Review. PubMed PMID: 17005598.

Clevers H. The cancer stem cell: premises, promises and challenges. Nat Med. 2011;17(3):313–9. https://doi.org/10.1038/nm.2304. Review. PubMed PMID: 21386835.

Cooper R, Sarioğlu S, Sökmen S, Füzün M, Küpelioğlu A, Valentine H, Görken IB, Airley R, West C. Glucose transporter-1 (GLUT-1): a potential marker of prognosis in rectal carcinoma? Br J Cancer. 2003;89(5):870–6. PubMed PMID: 12942120; PubMed Central PMCID: PMC2394489.

Demiral AN, Sarioglu S, Birlik B, Sen M, Kinay M. Prognostic significance of EGF receptor expression in early glottic cancer. Auris Nasus Larynx. 2004;31(4):417–24. PubMed PMID: 15571917.

Diepenbruck M, Christofori G. Epithelial-mesenchymal transition (EMT) and metastasis: yes, no, maybe? Curr Opin Cell Biol. 2016;43:7–13. https://doi.org/10.1016/j.ceb.2016.06.002. Review. PubMed PMID: 27371787.

Dikmen ZG, Ozgurtas T, Gryaznov SM, Herbert BS. Targeting critical steps of cancer metastasis and recurrence using telomerase template antagonists. Biochim Biophys Acta. 2009;1792(4):240–7. https://doi.org/10.1016/j.bbadis.2009.01.018. Review. PubMed PMID: 19419695.

Donnem T, Hu J, Ferguson M, Adighibe O, Snell C, Harris AL, Gatter KC, Pezzella F. Vessel co-option in primary human tumors and metastases: an obstacle to effective anti-angiogenic treatment? Cancer Med. 2013;2(4):427–36. https://doi.org/10.1002/cam4.105. Review. PubMed PMID: 24156015; PubMed Central PMCID: PMC3799277.

Folkman J, Merler E, Abernathy C, Williams G. Isolation of a tumor factor responsible for angiogenesis. J Exp Med. 1971;133(2):275–88. PubMed PMID: 4332371; PubMed Central PMCID: PMC2138906.

Gaggioli C, Hooper S, Hidalgo-Carcedo C, Grosse R, Marshall JF, Harrington K, Sahai E. Fibroblast-led collective invasion of carcinoma cells with differing roles for RhoGTPases in leading and following cells. Nat Cell Biol. 2007;9(12):1392–400. PubMed PMID: 18037882.

Gao H, Chakraborty G, Lee-Lim AP, Mo Q, Decker M, Vonica A, Shen R, Brogi E, Brivanlou AH, Giancotti FG. The BMP inhibitor Coco reactivates breast cancer cells at lung metastatic sites. Cell. 2012;150(4):764–79. https://doi.org/10.1016/j.cell.2012.06.035. Erratum in: Cell. 2012 Dec 7;151(6):1386–8. PubMed PMID: 22901808; PubMed Central PMCID: PMC3711709.

Giancotti FG. Mechanisms governing metastatic dormancy and reactivation. Cell. 2013;155(4):750–64. https://doi.org/10.1016/j.cell.2013.10.029. Review. PubMed PMID: 24209616; PubMed Central PMCID: PMC4354734.

Gilmore AP. Anoikis. Cell Death Differ. 2005;12(Suppl 2):1473–7. Review. PubMed PMID: 16247493.

Goldar S, Khaniani MS, Derakhshan SM, Baradaran B. Molecular mechanisms of apoptosis and roles in cancer development and treatment. Asian Pac J Cancer Prev. 2015;16(6):2129–44. Review. PubMed PMID: 25824729.

Granot Z, Henke E, Comen EA, King TA, Norton L, Benezra R. Tumor entrained neutrophils inhibit seeding in the premetastatic lung. Cancer Cell. 2011;20(3):300–14. https://doi.org/10.1016/j.ccr.2011.08.012. PubMed PMID: 21907922; PubMed Central PMCID: PMC3172582.

Greider CW, Blackburn EH. Identification of a specific telomere terminal transferase activity in Tetrahymena extracts. Cell. 1985;43(2 Pt 1):405–13. PubMed PMID: 3907856.

Greider CW, Blackburn EH. The telomere terminal transferase of Tetrahymena is a ribonucleoprotein enzyme with two kinds of primer specificity. Cell. 1987;51(6):887–98. PubMed PMID: 3319189.

Grigore AD, Jolly MK, Jia D, Farach-Carson MC, Levine H. Tumor budding: the name is EMT. Partial EMT. J Clin Med. 2016;5(5). pii: E51. doi: https://doi.org/10.3390/jcm5050051. Review. PubMed PMID: 27136592; PubMed Central PMCID: PMC4882480.

Gurel D, Ulukus Ç, Karasam V, Ellidokuz H, Umay C, Oztop İ, Sarioglu S. The prognostic value of morphologic findings for lung squamous cell carcinoma patients. Pathol Res Pract. 2016;212(1):1–9. https://doi.org/10.1016/j.prp.2015.10.006. PubMed PMID: 26608418.

Hanahan D, Weinberg RA. The hallmarks of cancer. Cell. 2000;100(1):57–70. Review. PubMed PMID: 10647931.

Hanahan D, Weinberg RA. Hallmarks of cancer: the next generation. Cell. 2011;144(5):646–74. https://doi.org/10.1016/j.cell.2011.02.013. Review. PubMed PMID: 21376230.

Hay ED. An overview of epithelio-mesenchymal transformation. Acta Anat (Basel). 1995;154(1):8–20. Review. PubMed PMID: 8714286.

Hurst DR, Welch DR. Metastasis suppressor genes at the interface between the environment and tumor cell growth. Int Rev Cell Mol Biol. 2011;286:107–80. https://doi.org/10.1016/B978-0-12-385859-7.00003-3. Review. PubMed PMID: 21199781; PubMed Central PMCID: PMC3575029.

Kabeya Y, Mizushima N, Ueno T, Yamamoto A, Kirisako T, Noda T, Kominami E, Ohsumi Y, Yoshimori T. LC3, a mammalian homologue of yeast Apg8p, is localized in autophagosome membranes after processing. EMBO J. 2000;19(21):5720–8.

Kalluri R, Weinberg RA. The basics of epithelial-mesenchymal transition. J Clin Invest. 2009;119(6):1420–8. https://doi.org/10.1172/JCI39104. Review. Erratum in: J Clin Invest. 2010 May 3;120(5):1786. PubMed PMID: 19487818; PubMed Central PMCID: PMC2689101.

Katsuragi Y, Ichimura Y, Komatsu M. p62/SQSTM1 functions as a signaling hub and an autophagy adaptor. FEBS J. 2015;282(24):4672–8. https://doi.org/10.1111/febs.13540. Review. PubMed PMID: 26432171.

Kerr JF, Wyllie AH, Currie AR. Apoptosis: a basic biological phenomenon with wide-ranging implications in tissue kinetics. Br J Cancer. 1972;26(4):239–57. Review. PubMed PMID: 4561027; PubMed Central PMCID: PMC2008650.

Kinugasa Y, Matsui T, Takakura N. CD44 expressed on cancer-associated fibroblasts is a functional molecule supporting the stemness and drug resistance of malignant cancer cells in the tumor microenvironment. Stem Cells. 2014;32(1):145–56. https://doi.org/10.1002/stem.1556. PubMed PMID: 24395741.

Kirimca F, Sarioglu S, Camsari T, Kavukçu S. Expression of CD44 and major histocompatibility complex class II antigens correlate with renal scarring in primary and systemic renal diseases. Scand J Urol Nephrol. 2001;35(6):509–14. PubMed PMID: 11848433.

Kreso A, Dick JE. Evolution of the cancer stem cell model. Cell Stem Cell. 2014;14(3):275–91. https://doi.org/10.1016/j.stem.2014.02.006. Review. PubMed PMID: 24607403.

Kumar V, Abas AK, Aster JC. eds. Robbins and Cotran pathologic basis of disease. 9th ed. Canada: Elsevier; 2015 p. 265–340.

Lambert AW, Pattabiraman DR, Weinberg RA. Emerging biological principles of metastasis. Cell. 2017;168(4):670–91. https://doi.org/10.1016/j.cell.2016.11.037. Review. PubMed PMID: 28187288; PubMed Central PMCID: PMC5308465.

Lee YK, Lee JA. Role of the mammalian ATG8/LC3 family in autophagy: differential and compensatory roles in the spatiotemporal regulation of autophagy. BMB Rep. 2016;49(8):424–30. Review. PubMed PMID: 27418283; PubMed Central PMCID: PMC5070729.

Lindahl T. My journey to DNA repair. Genomics Proteomics Bioinformatics. 2013;11(1):2–7. https://doi.org/10.1016/j.gpb.2012.12.001. Review. PubMed PMID: 23453014; PubMed Central PMCID: PMC4357663.

Lynch HT, Smyrk T. Hereditary nonpolyposis colorectal cancer (Lynch syndrome). An updated review. Cancer. 1996;78(6):1149–67. Review. PubMed PMID: 8826936.

Mancino M, Ametller E, Gascón P, Almendro V. The neuronal influence on tumor progression. Biochim Biophys Acta. 2011;1816(2):105–18. https://doi.org/10.1016/j.bbcan.2011.04.005. Review. PubMed PMID: 21616127.

Mapara MY, Sykes M. Tolerance and cancer: mechanisms of tumor evasion and strategies for breaking tolerance. J Clin Oncol. 2004;22(6):1136–51. Review. PubMed PMID: 15020616.

Millet C, Makovets S. Aneuploidy as a mechanism of adaptation to telomerase insufficiency. Curr Genet. 2016;62(3):557–64. https://doi.org/10.1007/s00294-015-0559-x. PubMed PMID: 26758992; PubMed Central PMCID: PMC4929173.

Modrich P. Mismatch repair, genetic stability, and cancer. Science. 1994;266(5193):1959–60. Review. PubMed PMID: 7801122.

Morgillo F, Della Corte CM, Fasano M, Ciardiello F. Mechanisms of resistance to EGFR-targeted drugs: lung cancer. ESMO Open. 2016;1(3):e000060. Review. PubMed PMID: 27843613; PubMed Central PMCID: PMC5070275.

Mowers EE, Sharifi MN, Macleod KF. Autophagy in cancer metastasis. Oncogene. 2016;36:1619–30. https://doi.org/10.1038/onc.2016.333. Review. PubMed PMID: 27593926.

Muenst S, Läubli H, Soysal SD, Zippelius A, Tzankov A, Hoeller S. The immune system and cancer evasion strategies: therapeutic concepts. J Intern Med. 2016;279(6):541–62. https://doi.org/10.1111/joim.12470. Review. PubMed PMID: 26748421.

Paoli P, Giannoni E, Chiarugi P. Anoikis molecular pathways and its role in cancer progression. Biochim Biophys Acta. 2013;1833(12):3481–98. https://doi.org/10.1016/j.bbamcr.2013.06.026. Review. PubMed PMID: 23830918.

Pattingre S, Espert L, Biard-Piechaczyk M, Codogno P. Regulation of macroautophagy by mTOR and Beclin 1 complexes. Biochimie. 2008;90(2):313–23. Review. PubMed PMID: 17928127.

Rybinski B, Franco-Barraza J, Cukierman E. The wound healing, chronic fibrosis, and cancer progression triad. Physiol Genomics. 2014;46(7):223–44. https://doi.org/10.1152/physiolgenomics.00158.2013. Review. PubMed PMID: 24520152; PubMed Central PMCID: PMC4035661.

Sahni S, Merlot AM, Krishan S, Jansson PJ, Richardson DR. Gene of the month:BECN1. J Clin Pathol. 2014;67(8):656–60. https://doi.org/10.1136/jclinpath-2014-202356. Review. PubMed PMID: 24811486.

Sancar A. DNA excision repair. Annu Rev Biochem. 1996;65:43–81. Review. Erratum in: Annu Rev Biochem 1997;66:VII. PubMed PMID: 8811174.

Sarioğlu S, Ozer E, Kirimca F, Sis B, Pabuççuoğlu U. Matrix metalloproteinase-2 expression in laryngeal preneoplastic and neoplastic lesions. Pathol Res Pract. 2001;197(7):483–6. PubMed PMID: 11482578.

Sarioglu S, Acara C, Akman FC, Dag N, Ecevit C, Ikiz AO, Cetinayak OH, Ada E, for Dokuz Eylül Head and Neck Tumour Group (DEHNTG). Tumor budding as a prognostic marker in laryngeal carcinoma. Pathol Res Pract. 2010;206(2):88–92. https://doi.org/10.1016/j.prp.2009.09.006. PubMed PMID: 19959297.

Sarioglu S, Dogan E, Sahin Y, Uzun E, Bekis R, Ada E, Sagol O, Akman F. Undifferentiated laryngeal carcinoma with pagetoid spread. Head Neck Pathol. 2016;10(2):252–5. https://doi.org/10.1007/s12105-015-0648-7. PubMed PMID: 26292650; PubMed Central PMCID: PMC4838975.

Sengiz S, Pabuççuoğlu U, Sarioğlu S. Immunohistological comparison of the World Health Organization (WHO) and Ljubljana classifications on the grading of preneoplastic lesions of the larynx. Pathol Res Pract. 2004;200(3):181–8. PubMed PMID: 15200269.

Sgambato A, Casaluce F, Sacco PC, Palazzolo G, Maione P, Rossi A, Ciardiello F, Gridelli C. Anti PD-1 and PDL-1 immunotherapy in the treatment of advanced non-small cell lung cancer (NSCLC): a review on toxicity profile and its management. Curr Drug Saf. 2016;11(1):62–8. Review. PubMed PMID: 26412670.

Sholl LM, Aisner DL, Allen TC, Beasley MB, Cagle PT, Capelozzi VL, Dacic S, Hariri LP, Kerr KM, Lantuejoul S, Mino-Kenudson M, Raparia K, Rekhtman N, Roy-Chowdhuri S, Thunnissen E, Tsao M, Vivero M, Yatabe Y. Liquid biopsy in lung cancer: a perspective from members of the Pulmonary Pathology Society. ArchPathol Lab Med. 2016;140(8):825–9. https://doi.org/10.5858/arpa.2016-0163-SA. PubMed PMID: 27195432.

Singh J, Hussain F, Decuzzi P. Role of differential adhesion in cell cluster evolution: from vasculogenesis to cancer metastasis. Comput Methods Biomech Biomed Engin. 2015;18(3):282–92. https://doi.org/10.1080/10255842.2013.792917. PubMed PMID: 23656190; PubMed Central PMCID: PMC3884055.

Sis B, Sağol O, Küpelioğlu A, Sokmen S, Terzi C, Fuzun M, Ozer E, Bishop P. Prognostic significance of matrix metalloproteinase-2, cathepsin D, and tenascin-C expression in colorectal carcinoma. Pathol Res Pract. 2004;200(5):379–87. PubMed PMID: 15239346.

Sis B, Sarioglu S, Sokmen S, Sakar M, Kupelioglu A, Fuzun M. Desmoplasia measured by computer assisted image analysis: an independent prognostic marker in colorectal carcinoma. J Clin Pathol. 2005;58(1):32–8. PubMed PMID: 15623479; PubMed Central PMCID: PMC1770537.

Snyder A, Makarov V, Merghoub T, Yuan J, Zaretsky JM, Desrichard A, Walsh LA, Postow MA, Wong P, Ho TS, Hollmann TJ, Bruggeman C, Kannan K, Li Y, Elipenahli C, Liu C, Harbison CT, Wang L, Ribas A, Wolchok JD, Chan TA. Genetic basis for clinical response to CTLA-4 blockade in melanoma. N Engl J Med. 2014;371(23):2189–99. https://doi.org/10.1056/NEJMoa1406498. PubMed PMID: 25409260; PubMed Central PMCID: PMC4315319.

Sökmen S, Lebe B, Sarioglu S, Füzün M, Terzi C, Küpelioglu A, Ellidokuz H. Prognostic value of CD44 expression in colorectal carcinomas. Anticancer Res. 2001a;21(6A):4121–6. PubMed PMID: 11911305.

Sökmen S, Sarioglu S, Füzün M, Terzi C, Küpelioglu A, Aslan B. Prognostic significance of angiogenesis in rectal cancer: a morphometric investigation. Anticancer Res. 2001b;21(6B):4341–8. PubMed PMID: 11908689.

Su Z, Yang Z, Xu Y, Chen Y, Yu Q. Apoptosis, autophagy, necroptosis, and cancer metastasis. Mol Cancer. 2015;14:48. https://doi.org/10.1186/s12943-015-0321-5. Review. PubMed PMID: 25743109; PubMed Central PMCID: PMC4343053.

Tataroglu C, Sarioglu S, Kargi A, Ozkal S, Aydin O. Fibrosis in Hodgkin and non-Hodgkin lymphomas. Pathol Res Pract. 2007;203(10):725–30. PubMed PMID: 17804176.

Tiwari N, Gheldof A, Tatari M, Christofori G. EMT as the ultimate survival mechanism of cancer cells. Semin Cancer Biol. 2012;22(3):194–207. https://doi.org/10.1016/j.semcancer.2012.02.013. Review. PubMed PMID: 22406545.

Topalian SL, Hodi FS, Brahmer JR, Gettinger SN, Smith DC, McDermott DF, Powderly JD, Carvajal RD, Sosman JA, Atkins MB, Leming PD, Spigel DR, Antonia SJ, Horn L, Drake CG,

Pardoll DM, Chen L, Sharfman WH, Anders RA, Taube JM, McMiller TL, Xu H, Korman AJ, Jure-Kunkel M, Agrawal S, McDonald D, Kollia GD, Gupta A, Wigginton JM, Sznol M. Safety, activity, and immune correlates of anti-PD-1 antibody in cancer. N Engl J Med. 2012;366(26):2443–54. https://doi.org/10.1056/NEJMoa1200690. PubMed PMID: 22658127; PubMed Central PMCID: PMC3544539.

Unlu M, Cetinayak HO, Onder D, Ecevit C, Akman F, Ikiz AO, Ada E, Karacali B, Sarioglu S. The prognostic value of tumor-stroma proportion in laryngeal squamous cell carcinoma. Turk Patoloji Derg. 2013;29(1):27–35. https://doi.org/10.5146/tjpath.2013.01144. PubMed PMID: 23354793.

Weber GF. Why does cancer therapy lack effective anti-metastasis drugs? Cancer Lett. 2013;328(2):207–11. https://doi.org/10.1016/j.canlet.2012.09.025. Review. PubMed PMID: 23059758.

West NP, Dattani M, McShane P, Hutchins G, Grabsch J, Mueller W, Treanor D, Quirke P, Grabsch H. The proportion of tumour cells is an independent predictor for survival in colorectal cancer patients. Br J Cancer. 2010;102(10):1519–23. https://doi.org/10.1038/sj.bjc.6605674. PubMed PMID: 20407439; PubMed Central PMCID: PMC2869173.

Wu ZZ, Zhang JJ, Gao CC, Zhao M, Liu SY, Gao GM, Zheng ZH. Expression of autophagy related genes mTOR, Becline-1, LC3 and p62 in the peripheral blood mononuclear cells of systemic lupus erythematosus. Am J Clin Exp Immunol. 2017;6(1):1–8. PubMed PMID: 28123902; PubMed Central PMCID: PMC5259582.

Yamaguchi H, Sakai R. Direct interaction between carcinoma cells and cancer associated fibroblasts for the regulation of cancer invasion. Cancers (Basel). 2015;7(4):2054–62. https://doi.org/10.3390/cancers7040876. Review. PubMed PMID: 26473929; PubMed Central PMCID: PMC4695876.

Yan Y, Zuo X, Wei D. Concise review: emerging role of CD44 in cancer stem cells: a promising biomarker and therapeutic target. Stem Cells Transl Med. 2015;4(9):1033–43. https://doi.org/10.5966/sctm.2015-0048. Review. PubMed PMID: 26136504; PubMed Central PMCID: PMC4542874.

Yu M, Bardia A, Wittner BS, Stott SL, Smas ME, Ting DT, Isakoff SJ, Ciciliano JC, Wells MN, Shah AM, Concannon KF, Donaldson MC, Sequist LV, Brachtel E, Sgroi D, Baselga J, Ramaswamy S, Toner M, Haber DA, Maheswaran S. Circulating breast tumor cells exhibit dynamic changes in epithelial and mesenchymal composition. Science. 2013;339(6119):580–4. https://doi.org/10.1126/science.1228522. PubMed PMID: 23372014; PubMed Central PMCID: PMC3760262.

Zhou W, Yuan J. Necroptosis in health and diseases. Semin Cell Dev Biol. 2014;35:14–23. https://doi.org/10.1016/j.semcdb.2014.07.013. Review. PubMed PMID: 25087983.

Zwaans BM, Bielenberg DR. Potential therapeutic strategies for lymphatic metastasis. Microvasc Res. 2007;74(2–3):145–58. Review. PubMed PMID:17950368; PubMed Central PMCID: PMC2525453.

Tumor Deposits; Mechanisms, Morphology, and Differential Diagnosis

2

Morphology and Differential Diagnosis of Free Tumor Deposits

Tumor deposits may be named as satellites or extramural tumor extensions for colorectal carcinoma cases. The morphological features of these lesions, the "free tumor deposits," are described as follows according to the 2013 classification of the College of American Pathologists (CAP): tumor deposits or satellites are tumor nodules with regular or irregular contours, located away from the primary tumor mass, but within the lymphatic draining area, devoid of the morphological features of a lymph node (http://www.cap.org/ShowProperty?nodePath=/UCMCon/Contribution%20Folders/WebContent/pdf/colon-13protocol-3300.pdf. Accessed 24 March 2017). This type of tumor nodules were described by Gabriel WB et al. in 1935 (Gabriel et al. 1935). Tumor deposits may be seen in association with lymphatics, nerves, or vessels; they may either have regular or irregular contours (Ueno et al. 2012). Host reactions to the primary tumors may be seen surrounding the tumor deposits including inflammation and desmoplasia.

The tumor deposits are also recognized by pathologists according to the information at the 7th edition of the American Joint Committee on Cancer (AJCC) classification: "discrete foci of tumor found in the pericolic or perirectal fat or in adjacent mesentery (mesocolic fat) away from the leading edge of the tumor and showing no evidence of residual lymph node tissue" (Sobin et al. 2009).

The most important differential diagnosis of tumor deposits is between these lesions and the metastatic lymph nodes, the ones with extranodal invasion in particular (Figs. 2.1, 2.2, 2.3, and 2.4). It may be speculated that any tumor deposit had once been a metastatic lymph node with extensive tumor growth, replacing any component of a lymph node (Fig. 2.5). Previously, especially for the colorectal carcinomas, tumor deposits were classified as metastatic lymph nodes if they had smooth contours and named as vascular invasion in case they had irregular contours and they had been related to the T stage (Ueno et al. 2012; Rock et al. 2014). However, the 7th edition of the UICC classification accepted these masses as tumor deposits, allowing their recognition as distinct tumor structures. Although the discussions about the N staging in association with tumor deposits are ongoing, now they are better recognized morphologically.

© Springer International Publishing AG 2018
S. Sarioglu, *Tumor Deposits*, https://doi.org/10.1007/978-3-319-68582-3_2

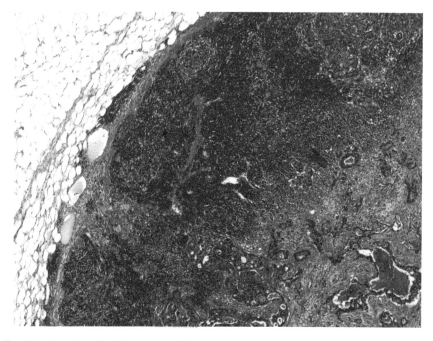

Fig. 2.1 Lymph node with preserved lymph node capsule, sinuses, and lymphoid follicles replaced by an adenocarcinoma forming complex glandular structures. The neoplastic structures are surrounded by a desmoplastic stroma. All the pathologists would agree that this is a metastatic lymph node (H&E, Original magnification ×10)

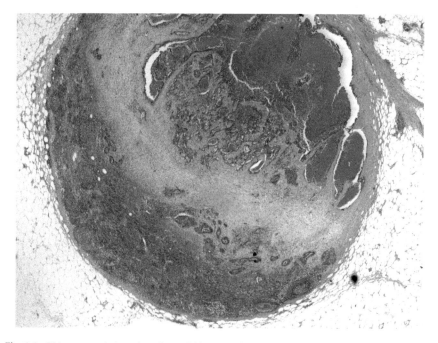

Fig. 2.2 This metastatic lymph node would increase the κ value if it was included at a set prepared for interobserver agreement (H&E, Original magnification ×4)

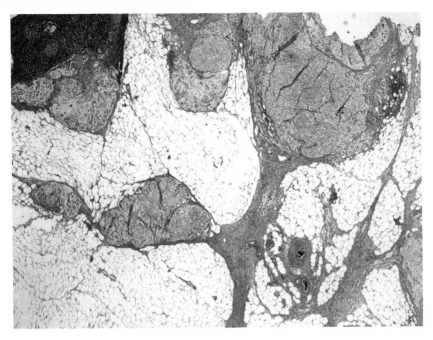

Fig. 2.3 At the left top, a metastatic lymph node is easy to identify, and the other irregular tumor groups seem to be tumor deposits; however, it is not very easy to count them; in this case the tumor was a signet-ring cell carcinoma (H&E, Original magnification ×10)

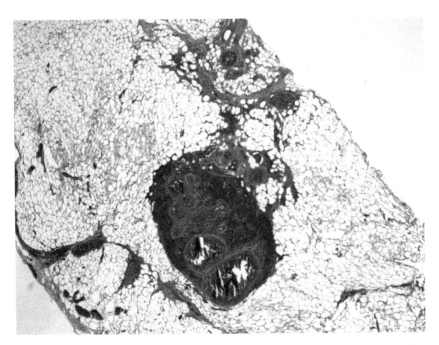

Fig. 2.4 This metastatic lymph node seems to have perinodal invasion; however, the adjacent malignant glandular structures at the upper part of the image may be perivascular tumor deposits (H&E, Original magnification ×2)

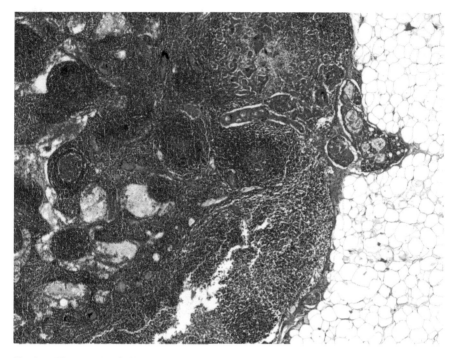

Fig. 2.5 The capsule of this metastatic lymph node is being invaded by the adenocarcinoma. In case it was extensive, leading to the total replacement of the lymph node with extranodal invasion, it could lead to a diagnostic difficulty between a tumor deposit and metastatic lymph node (H&E, Original magnification ×10)

The interobserver agreement about the tumor deposits was evaluated in a series of 25 difficult images by Rock et al. (2014). A group of gastrointestinal pathologists were asked to evaluate these cases, and the images were presented in the article. The morphologic features, a distinctly thick capsule, peripheral lymphoid follicles, peripheral lymphoid rim, and size >3 mm, were used for distinguishing a tumor mass as a metastatic lymph node by most of the participants. Deep sectioning may reveal lymph node structures allowing proper classification (Fig. 2.6). At the selected difficult 25 cases in the series by Rock JB, the κ statistic was found to be 0.48, reflecting moderate agreement between pathologists. In the series by Ueno et al. (2012), the extramural tumor lesions were evaluated by 11 observers, and the interobserver agreement was substantial ($\kappa = 0.74$), in randomly selected cases.

Clinical Relevance of Free Tumor Deposits

Cancer-related deaths are of utmost importance all around the world. Prognostic and predictive markers are being constantly sought for, for nearly all types of carcinomas. Tumor, lymph node, and distant metastasis stage groups are the best-categorized, evidence-based prognostic factors for many types of carcinomas.

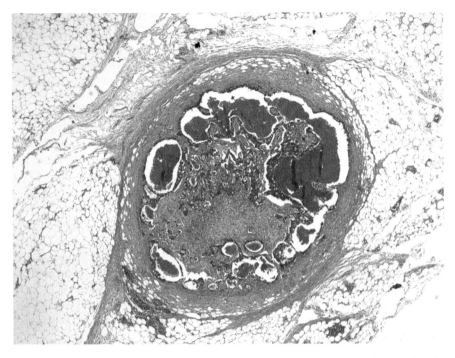

Fig. 2.6 This tumor nodule has smooth contours, but it has no other features of a lymph node. Considering the strong desmoplasia at the central part, fibrotic reaction at the periphery should not be unexpected. There is not much evidence to name this lesion as a metastatic lymph node, so it seems this is a smooth contoured tumor deposit (H&E, Original magnification ×10)

The importance of TDs in tumor progression and prognosis did not attract any interest for a significant period of time after the first report about them in 1935. However, their association with poor prognosis was reported in different series during the last two decades (Ueno et al. 1998; Ratto et al. 2002) with an impact factor leading to changes in TNM classification for colorectal cancer in 2009 at the 7th edition (Sobin et al. 2009). Cases without lymph node metastasis, but with tumor deposits, were classified as pathological node stage 1c (pN1c), but the N stage does not differ if a case have metastatic lymph nodes, with tumor deposits.

This classification has been criticized as it only considered TDs in the absence of lymph node metastasis. The shape/type, number, and diameter of the deposits do not change the N stage at the present for colorectal carcinomas. In a meta-analysis by Nagtegaal et al. (2017), 10,106 patients were analyzed. It was shown that the cases with TDs had the worst outcome in this series, whether there was lymph node metastasis or not. Furthermore, if the number of TDs was more than 2 and the diameter more than 12 mm, the prognosis was significantly worse.

At the 8th edition of the TNM classification in 2017, the criteria for TDs were changed as follows: tumor deposits should not have histological evidence of residual lymph node or identifiable vascular or neural structures. If a vessel wall is identifiable on H&E or other stains, it should be classified as either venous (V1/2) or lymphatic invasion (LI). If neural structures are identifiable, the lesion should be classified as perineural invasion (PNI). Tumor deposits do not change the primary tumor T category, but change the node status (N) to N1c if all regional lymph nodes are negative on pathological examination.

TDs are not confined to the colorectal carcinomas, but they are also identified in gastric carcinomas. They are associated with poor prognosis also for the gastric carcinomas, but the studies in gastric carcinomas are sparse compared with the colorectal carcinomas (Sun et al. 2012, Liebig et al. 2013, Ersen et al. 2014).

The tumor deposits are not confined to the gastrointestinal system, and they may be identified in head and neck tumors (Jose et al. 2004; Sarioglu et al. 2016a). In a series of 140 head and neck squamous cell carcinomas, we have found TDs in 17% of the cases, and only tumor deposits were significant for survival, increasing the risk of death from disease 3.4 times (Sarioglu et al. 2016a).

This short summary highlights the existence of TDs in different organs and in different types of malignant tumors such as adenocarcinomas and squamous cell carcinomas. Other types of carcinomas use similar pathways during metastasis like lymph node metastasis and distant metastasis. Probably other types of carcinomas may also share the same pathways that lead to the formation of TDs.

The morphological and clinical features of TDs are mostly described and discussed in colorectal carcinomas. For TDs arising from other organs and other types of carcinomas, there are very few reports.

Basically, this chapter will focus on the mechanisms of the formation of the TDs.

Mechanisms of Tumor Deposit Formation

Tumor deposits observed at the extramural region of the colorectal or gastric regions or at the lymph node dissection specimens of the head and neck give rise to questions about the routes of dissemination. How do malignant cells travel to this area? At the College of American Pathologists, the mechanism is briefly defined as "Most examples are due to lymphovascular or, more rarely, perineural invasion" (http://www.cap.org/ShowProperty?nodePath=/UCMCon/Contribution%20Folders/WebContent/pdf/colon-13protocol-3300.pdf. Accessed 24 Mar 2017).

The morphological clues of these deposits led to some hypothesis about these routes. The tumor deposits may be seen surrounding a peripheral nerve, or it may be adjacent to a nerve. In other cases, they may be associated with a lymphatic or blood vessel. In some instances, three structures, blood vessels, lymphatics, and nerves, are closely packed and so is the tumor deposit not allowing the distinction of the predominant association. Furthermore, for some of the deposits, none of these structures are observed at the vicinity.

In a research article by Ueno et al. (2012), the TDs were morphologically grouped into vascular/perineural groups and tumor nodules. These morphological classification attempts were evaluated for prognostic implications, along with T and N categories, which are very important for the patient management. However, as we concentrate on the tumor progression mechanisms through tumor deposits at this session, we will focus on the mechanism of tumor extension with each mechanism.

Neurotrophic Extravascular Migratory Metastasis, Perineural Invasion, and Perineural-Type Tumor Deposit Formation

Nerves are surrounded by a sheath made up of three layers: the epineurium, the perineurium, and the endoneurium. These structures are made up of collagen bundles and basement membrane material which are not easy to invade. The vasa nervorum and the perineural lymphatic channels are located at the outer zone surrounding the epineurium (Liebig et al. 2013).

Perineural area is an alternative pathway for tumor dissemination, and this is one of the routes of extravascular migratory metastasis (Lugassy et al. 2014). Perineural invasion can be identified during light microscopic examination of the tissue sections. The positivity rates increase with the application of immunohistochemical staining with antibodies like S100 which is positive at the peripheral nerves as well as double immunostaining with S100 and an epithelial marker (Zhou et al. 2014). Perineural invasion is not mutually exclusive for carcinomas; it was also identified in prostate tissue devoid of cancer, and the perineural cells were prostatic glands.

In carcinoma cases, the definition for histopathological diagnosis of PNI raised a lot of debate. There may be different histological appearances; sometimes the tumor cells are located within the peripheral nerve. Sometimes they are seen surrounding the peripheral nerve. In these cases, the diagnosis is straightforward. However, it is hard to be sure of PNI, in case only a few cells are observed at the perineural area or in case the peripheral nerve section is in the tumor. It was suggested that, if more than one third of the nerve is surrounded by the tumor cells, PNI should be diagnosed (Liebig et al. 2013).

Experimental studies demonstrated that there is a movement toward the ganglia of the tumor cells and growth of neurites toward neurotropic cancer colonies (Ayala et al. 2001). In case a similar experimental system was enriched with stromal cells, increased neurites and cancer colonies were observed (Cornell et al. 2003). These results highlight the interaction of tumor cells and nerves as well as stromal cells during PNI. Increased expression of neurotrophins was identified both by the tumor cells and the neural cells during PNI (Ketterer et al. 2003; Figs. 2.7 and 2.8). Neurotrophins are among the neurotrophic factor family members which are important in different types of carcinomas during tumor progression and prognosis; they include the following factors:

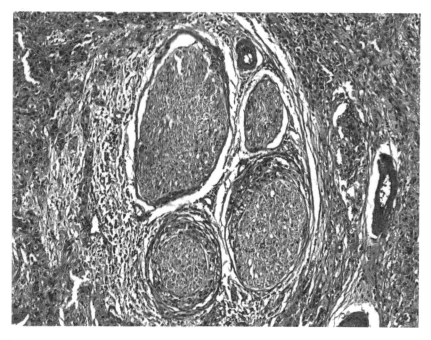

Fig. 2.7 Malignant cells surrounding the peripheral nerves: "perineural invasion". Note the enlarged peripheral nerves and thick groups of malignant cells surrounding these bundles, probably nourishing eachother by growth factors (H&E, Original magnification, ×20)

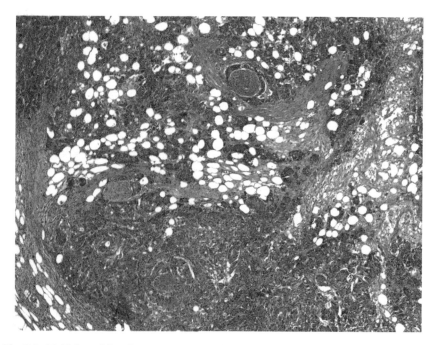

Fig. 2.8 Multiple peripheral nerves are surrounded by perineural invasion, and there is irregular tumor deposit formation (H&E, Original magnification ×4)

– Neurotrophins
– Neuropoietins
– Insulin-like growth factor
– Transforming growth factor
– Fibroblast growth factors
– Other growth factors (Mancino 2011)

Neurotrophins are among the factors important for perineural tumor growth during cancer progression and they include the ones listed:

– Nerve growth factor (NGF)
– Brain-derived neurotrophic factor (BDNF)
– Neurotrophin 3 (NT-3)
– Neurotrophin 4/5 (NT-4/NT-5)
– Glial cell line-derived neurotrophic factor (GDNF) (Liebig et al. 2013)
– Novel neurotrophin 1 (Mancino 2011)

Like in many steps in cancer progression and invasion, proteases are important during perineural tumor growth. MMP2 and MMP9 are important in PNI. Interestingly the nerve growth factors like NGF and GDNF were found to increase MMP expression, further increasing the perineural growth. Invasion of the basement membrane is a primary step in cancer progression from in situ carcinoma to invasive carcinoma. Basement membrane material is also a component of the perineural region, and its invasion by the tumor cells is increased with the nerve growth factors, BDNF, NT-3, as well as NGF, according to experimental models (Liebig et al. 2013).

Chemokines, a family of small soluble proteins, are important in cell migration. The signaling axis of chemokine (C-C motif) ligand 2 (CCL-2) and its receptor (CCR2) was identified as an important step in PNI in prostatic carcinoma. The possibility of treatment of carcinoma patients with PNI by CCR2 antagonists may prove fruitful (He et al. 2015).

Some types of carcinomas are recognized with their neurotropism, like the adenoid cystic carcinomas of the salivary glands and seromucinous glands. In a meta-analysis including 1332 patients, the ratio of the cases with PNI was 43.2% (Ju et al. 2016). This may be different for other types of carcinomas like the adenocarcinomas of the colorectal region; in a systematic review including 22,900 patients, the ratio of PNI-positive cases was 18.2%. However, in any case the poor prognostic impact of PNI is constant in nearly all types of carcinomas like the two types mentioned above (Knijn et al. 2016). Although the tumor deposits may be seen adjacent to the neural structures away from the tumor mass, the positivity of tumor deposits is not related to the positivity of perineural invasion in different series (Ersen et al. 2014; Sarioglu et al. 2016a). This may be due to the other mechanisms of tumor deposit formation like the perivascular and perilymphatic routes. However, in the series of gastric carcinomas by Ersen A et al., the incidence of perineural invasion was 61%, and the ratio of tumor deposit positive cases was 23%, but perineural-type tumor deposit was observed only in 1% of the cases and 13% of the cases had tumor deposits of mixed types. In any case perineural invasion is much frequent than tumor deposit formation.

What is the trigger for the tumor deposit formation during their voyage at the perineural region? During the intravascular metastatic pathway, the epithelial cells are thought to stop proliferation, but when they extravasate, they don't always immediately start proliferation leading to tumor dormancy. Many factors were described for the activation of tumor cell proliferation or the endurance of the dormancy (Gao et al. 2012; Giancotti 2013). However, we are devoid of such information for the malignant cells which invade the perineural space.

Angiotrophic Extravascular Migratory Metastasis and Perivascular-Type Tumor Deposit Formation

Perivascular tumor deposits may be related to circulating tumor cells, which end up with metastasis at the site of the tumor deposit. However, morphological features give rise to questions about extravascular spread as an alternative or the main mechanism.

Extravascular migratory metastasis (EVMM) is a mechanism of tumor spread best defined in malignant melanoma. During this journey, melanoma cells act like pericytes and replace these cells. The angiotrophic malignant tumor cells adhere to the abluminal surface of the vessels and travel to distant sites without entering the vascular channels. The speed of the spread of the cells was measured as 0.1–2 μm/min, resulting in 5.2–105 cm/year. Melanoma cells originate from the neural crest, and EVMM shares many properties with neural cell migration. The melanoblasts originating from the dorsal neural tube take the dorsolateral pathway to reach and home to the skin for population. During development, the mechanisms of this migration include the same steps with EVMM. This points to a regressive phenotype of melanoma cells mimicking embryogenesis during EVMM. However, melanocytes are not the only cells who use this pathway; neurons, glial, smooth muscle, and connective tissue cells are among the others. Namely, during metastases of melanoma with this mechanism, the steps are as follows:

- Single tumor cell at the invasive border of the tumor probably with stem cell features
- Angiotropism
- Epithelial-mesenchymal transition with pericytic mimicry
- Perivascular migration
- Repopulation to form metastasis (Lugassy et al. 2014)

Melanoma cells are derived from the neural crest, as they arise from the melanocytes which travel to the skin and mucosa during embryogenesis from the neural crest, and some authors describe this process as type I epithelial-mesenchymal transition (EMT) (Kalluri and Weinberg 2009). It is suggested that, due to this ability, melanoma cells do not have to have classical EMT for metastasis; rather they undergo an "EMT-like process." Changes in some phenotypical markers are observed during metastasis, like the decrease in ZEB2 and Slug which are characteristics of differentiated melanoma cells and ZEB1 and Twist which are markers of the invasive phenotype.

There have been some differences between the metastatic patterns of malignant melanoma; while the primary tumors at the head and neck region and lower extremities cause in satellite or in-transit metastasis, 30% of the malignant melanomas of the upper extremity and trunk give rise to distant metastasis (Adler et al. 2017).

Satellite metastasis is a well-recognized mechanism of melanoma spread. It is a metastatic nodule within two centimeters to the main tumor. The in-transit metastasis is the development of metastatic nodule/nodules, between the first draining lymph node (sentinel lymph node) and the tumor, within the dermal and subepidermal lymphatics (Adler et al. 2017). In a series by Mervic (2012), including 9044 malignant melanoma cases, female patients developed earlier metastasis, more frequently as satellite nodules, than male patients who developed earlier metastasis to the lymph nodes; however, the time to distant metastasis and overall survival were worse for the male patients. In the series of malignant melanoma cases by Wilmott et al. (2012), angiotropism was identified as one of the independent predictive factors for tumor deposit formation along with Clark level, absence of regression, and acral location.

There may be three factors that should be addressed about the similarities or differences between malignant melanomas and carcinomas, and there is rather sparse information about these mechanisms in literature. While the CAP protocol describes tumor deposits synonyms with satellites, their relation with the mechanism of melanoma spread is obscure (http://www.cap.org/ShowProperty?nodePath=/UCMCon/Contribution%20Folders/WebContent/pdf/colon-13protocol-3300.pdf. Accessed 24 March 2017; Bentolila et al. 2016):

1. Although the literature about tumor deposit formation in carcinomas is expanding, tumor deposit formation in malignant melanomas is not described previously to the best of our knowledge. From a mechanistic view, can malignant melanoma satellite nodules or in-transit metastasis be accepted as tumor deposits? The in-transit metastasis may represent this phenomenon at least partially. Were the radical lymph node dissection materials ever evaluated for tumor deposits? In fact, we have head and neck malignant melanoma cases with neck metastasis with the unequivocal morphology of tumor deposits.
2. The information about the perivascular invasion of the carcinoma cells is also sparse; however, the histopathological evaluation of the carcinomas allows the observation of unequivocal perivascular invasion. Comparison of the images for angiotropism of malignant melanoma with cases of carcinomas may be helpful. The images for angiotropism in malignant melanoma series presented small and thin vessels, while the carcinoma cases may have perivascular invasion of much larger vessels (Figs. 2.9, 2.10, and 2.11). Is the mechanism of invasion with "angiotropism" a relevant mechanism for carcinomas?
3. Considering malignant melanoma cells derivation from the neural crest, and embryological tendency to act in an EMT-like fashion, what might be similarities and/or differences between melanoma and carcinoma cells during perivascular invasion?

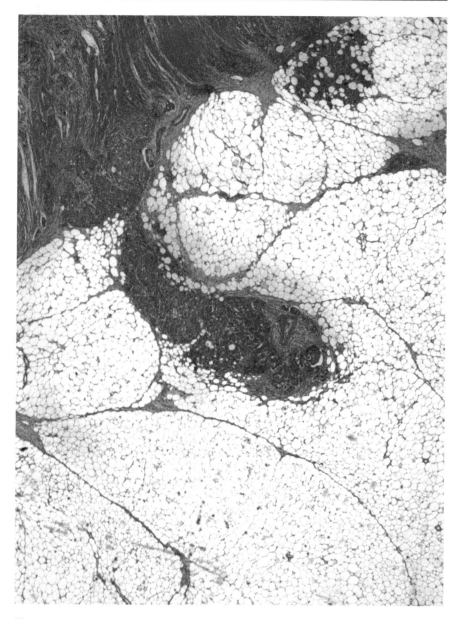

Fig. 2.9 In this case, the tumor spread from the main tumor mass like a tongue from the muscularis propria into the surrounding fat tissue. The perpendicular growth pattern and the vascular structure at the base of the invasive mass seem to be related to the perivascular invasion (H&E, Original magnification ×4)

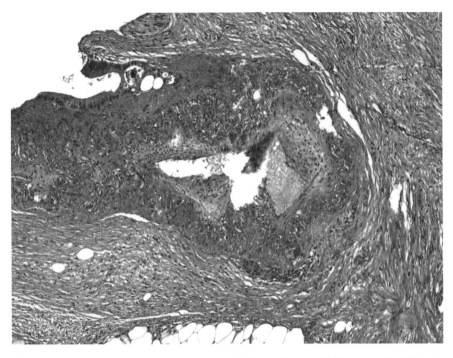

Fig. 2.10 This vessel is surrounded by tumor cells. The malignant cells have a poorly differentiated morphology at the bottom right, and at the top left, they form a well-formed glandular structure. The tumor invasion seems to be at the outer muscular layer of the vessel. Tumors forming
glandular structures during this process; probably angiotrophic extravascular migratory metastasis
may be well or poorly differentiated. Note the distinctly thickened vessel wall. Like the neural
growth factors influencing the peripheral nerves to get thickened, vessels with perivascular invasion are also very thick walled (H&E, Original magnification ×40)

Considering the perivascular route, the pathway may resemble an "allocated
highway" allowing the escape from the immune surveillance (Sarioglu et al. 2016a),
but during migration through this space, the tumor cells still require many properties and need the proper adhesion molecules and matrix metalloproteinases. Actually
the space where they are traveling is not really a "space" as it is very frequently
named as, but it is another part of the human organism with extracellular matrix and
connective tissue components.

Tumor Deposits Associated with Lymphatics

If the lymphatics are iterated at the histopathological sections, it may be seen that
there are lymphocyte groups surrounding the lymphatics but not forming lymph
nodes. These might be sites for lymphatic extravasation both for the lymphocytes
and for the malignant cells (Figs. 2.12 and 2.13).

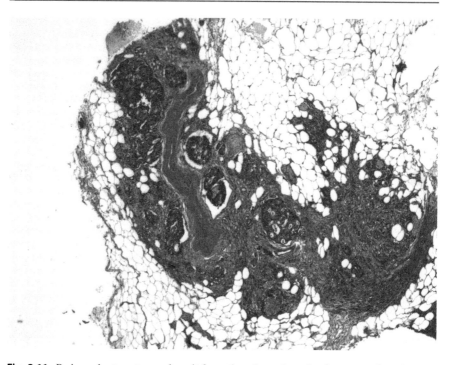

Fig. 2.11 Perivascular-type tumor deposit formation, the end result of extravascular migratory metastasis; note the irregular contours of the tumor deposit (H&E, Original magnification ×4)

Like the perineural and perivascular tumor deposits, perilymphatic tumor deposits may be recognized during histopathological evaluation. The tumor deposits with regular contours seem to be more frequently associated with lymphatics. However, unlike perineural and perivascular spread, there is not much information about perilymphatic spread. As the lymphatic vessels are different from the blood vessels, like they do not have pericytes or basement membranes at the distal ends, it is easier for the tumor cells to invade the lymphatics, and probably the extravasation process is also easier. Increased interstitial pressure induces the opening of the "button junctions." Both the lack of layers surrounding the lymphatics and button junctions allows easier access of the tumor cells to the lymphatic tumor compared with an arterial structure (Baluk et al. 2007). Any tumor cells extravasating at sites other than the lymph nodes will result in a tumor deposit, if they overcome dormancy, survive, and proliferate. They will form a tumor mess devoid of the capsule of the lymph node which is still a barrier for further spread (Figs. 2.14).

Other Routes of Tumor Spread

Tumors find even more routes for dissemination. One of these is by the invasion of skin adnexal structures named as *adnexotropism* targeting hair follicles and sweat

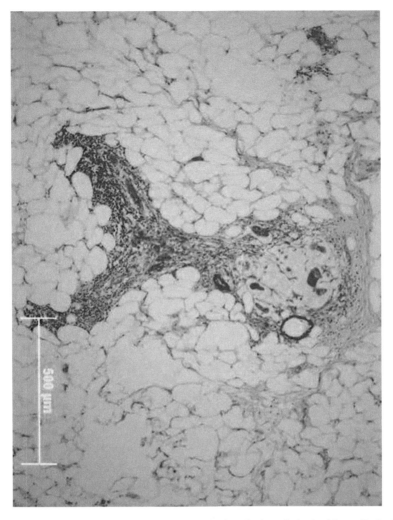

Fig. 2.12 A group of lymphocytes surrounding the lymphatics admixed with small glandular structures, which are in fact malignant, from an adenocarcinoma of colon. These small neoplastic cell groups may grow into a tumor deposit. Note the lymphocytes are not arranged at a lymph node. It seems the neoplastic cells arrive to this site and extravasate to form deposits instead of a lymph node (H&E, Original magnification ×10)

glands. The peritoneum and pleura may be a pathway for the spread. Brain ventricles, the choroid plexus, and glia limitans may also serve the spreading purpose of the tumor cells. Collagen fibers, bone cavities, and any structure surrounded by a basement membrane may form a pathway for tumor dissemination (Bentolila et al. 2016). Pagetoid spread is related to adnexotropism in some cases, and intraductal spread along the salivary gland duct was proposed for cases arising from the salivary glands (Sarioglu et al. 2016b); however, this cannot explain all the scenarios.

Possible mechanisms of tumor deposit formation are presented in Fig. 2.15.

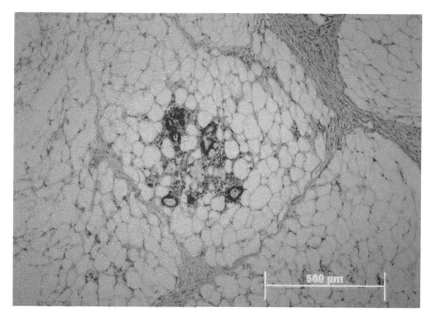

Fig. 2.13 Small group of malignant glandular cells surrounded by few lymphocytes. These might have arrived through intralymphatic pathway and extravasated at this point. Note the lack of nerves and blood vessels, allowing another indirect proof for the importance of lymphatics, which are not easily detected in H&E sections (H&E, Original magnification ×10)

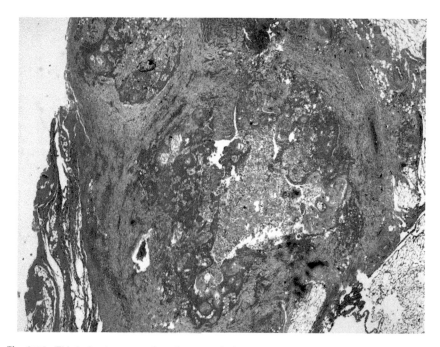

Fig. 2.14 This lesion is a tumor deposit metastatic from a squamous cell carcinoma with irregular contours. There are a few thick-walled vessels at the right side. It is hard to classify this lesion as perivascular, perineural, or lymphatic (H&E, Original magnification ×10)

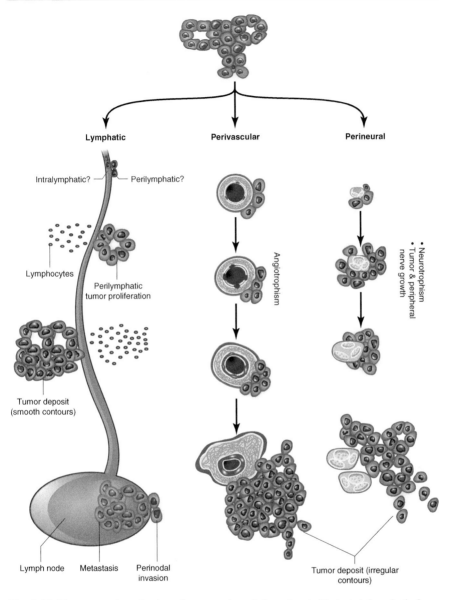

Fig. 2.15 The proposed mechanisms for tumor deposit formation is illustrated; lymphatic forming deposits with smooth contours, perineural or perivascular invasion, and spread forming deposits with irregular contours. During the extramural spread, the tumor does not have to grow gradually. In most of the cases, probably malignant cells travel/grow surrounding the perineural or perivascular space as a thin layer of few cells. In this illustration, lymph node metastasis seems to be distal to the tumor deposit formation. However, we do not know if this is true for the carcinomas

References

Adler NR, Haydon A, McLean CA, Kelly JW, Mar VJ. Metastatic pathways in patients with cutaneous melanoma. Pigment Cell Melanoma Res. 2017;30(1):13–27. https://doi.org/10.1111/pcmr.12544. Review. PubMed PMID: 27900851.

Ayala GE, Wheeler TM, Shine HD, et al. In vitro dorsal root ganglia and human prostate cell line interaction: redefining perineural invasion in prostate cancer. Prostate. 2001;49:213–23.

Baluk P, Fuxe J, Hashizume H, Romano T, Lashnits E, Butz S, Vestweber D, Corada M, Molendini C, Dejana E, McDonald DM. Functionally specialized junctions between endothelial cells of lymphatic vessels. J Exp Med. 2007;204(10):2349–62. PubMed PMID: 17846148; PubMed Central PMCID: PMC2118470.

Bentolila LA, Prakash R, Mihic-Probst D, Wadehra M, Kleinman HK, Carmichael TS, Péault B, Barnhill RL, Lugassy C. Imaging of angiotropism/vascular co-option in a murine model of brain melanoma: implications for melanoma progression along extravascular pathways. Sci Rep. 2016;6:23834. https://doi.org/10.1038/srep23834. PubMed PMID: 27048955; PubMed Central PMCID: PMC4822155.

Cornell RJ, Rowley D, Wheeler T, et al. Neuroepithelial interactions in prostate cancer are enhanced in the presence of prostatic stroma. Urology. 2003;61:870–5.

Ersen A, Unlu MS, Akman T, Sagol O, Oztop I, Atila K, Bora S, Ellidokuz H, Sarioglu S. Tumor deposits in gastric carcinomas. Pathol Res Pract. 2014;210(9):565–70. https://doi.org/10.1016/j.prp.2014.03.006. PubMed PMID: 24726262.

Gabriel WB, Dukes CE, Bussey HJR. Lymphatic spread in cancer of the rectum. Br J Surg. 1935;23:395–413.

Gao H, Chakraborty G, Lee-Lim AP, Mo Q, Decker M, Vonica A, Shen R, Brogi E, Brivanlou AH, Giancotti FG. The BMP inhibitor Coco reactivates breast cancer cells at lung metastatic sites. Cell. 2012;150(4):764–79. https://doi.org/10.1016/j.cell.2012.06.035. Erratum in: Cell. 2012 Dec 7;151(6):1386–8. PubMed PMID: 22901808; PubMed Central PMCID: PMC3711709.

Giancotti FG. Mechanisms governing metastatic dormancy and reactivation. Cell. 2013;155(4):750–64. https://doi.org/10.1016/j.cell.2013.10.029. Review. PubMed PMID: 24209616; PubMed Central PMCID: PMC4354734.

He S, He S, Chen CH, Deborde S, Bakst RL, Chernichenko N, McNamara WF, Lee SY, Barajas F, Yu Z, Al-Ahmadie HA, Wong RJ. The chemokine (CCL2-CCR2) signaling axis mediates perineural invasion. Mol Cancer Res. 2015;13(2):380–90. https://doi.org/10.1158/1541-7786. MCR-14-0303. PubMed PMID: 25312961; PubMed Central PMCID: PMC4336839.

http://www.cap.org/ShowProperty?nodePath=/UCMCon/Contribution%20Folders/WebContent/pdf/colon-13protocol-3300.pdf. Accessed 24 Mar 2017.

Jose J, Moor JW, Coatesworth AP, Johnston C, MacLennan K. Soft tissue deposits in neck dissections of patients with head and neck squamous cell carcinoma: prospective analysis of prevalence, survival, and its implications. Arch Otolaryngol Head Neck Surg. 2004;130(2):157–60. PubMed PMID: 14967743.

Ju J, Li Y, Chai J, Ma C, Ni Q, Shen Z, Wei J, Sun M. The role of perineural invasion on head and neck adenoid cystic carcinoma prognosis: a systematic review and meta-analysis. Oral Surg Oral Med Oral Pathol Oral Radiol. 2016;122(6):691–701. https://doi.org/10.1016/j.oooo.2016.08.008. Review. PubMed PMID: 27727107.

Kalluri R, Weinberg RA. The basics of epithelial-mesenchymal transition. J Clin Invest. 2009;119(6):1420–8. https://doi.org/10.1172/JCI39104. Review. Erratum in: J Clin Invest. 2010 May 3;120(5):1786. PubMed PMID: 19487818; PubMed Central PMCID: PMC2689101.

Ketterer K, Rao S, Friess H, et al. Reverse transcription PCR analysis of laser-captured cells points to potential paracrine and autocrine actions of neurotrophins in pancreatic cancer. Clin Cancer Res. 2003;9:5127–36.

Knijn N, Mogk SC, Teerenstra S, Simmer F, Nagtegaal ID. Perineural invasion is a strong prognostic factor in colorectal cancer: a systematic review. Am J Surg Pathol. 2016;40(1):103–12. https://doi.org/10.1097/PAS.0000000000000518. Review. PubMed PMID: 26426380.

Liebig C, Ayala G, Wilks JA, Lee HS, Lee HE, Yang HK, Kim WH. Perigastric tumor deposits in primary gastric cancer: implications for patient prognosis and staging. Ann Surg Oncol. 2013;20(5):1604–13. https://doi.org/10.1245/s10434-012-2692-9. PubMed PMID: 23184289.

Lugassy C, Zadran S, Bentolila LA, Wadehra M, Prakash R, Carmichael ST, Kleinman HK, Péault B, Larue L, Barnhill RL. Angiotropism, pericytic mimicry and extravascular migratory metastasis in melanoma: an alternative to intravascular cancer dissemination. Cancer Microenviron. 2014;7(3):139–52. https://doi.org/10.1007/s12307-014-0156-4. PubMed PMID: 25304454; PubMed Central PMCID: PMC4275501.

Mancino M, Ametller E, Gascón P, Almendro V. The neuronal influence on tumor progression. Biochimica et Biophysica Acta (BBA) - Reviews on Cancer. 2011;1816(2):105–118.

Mervic L. Time course and pattern of metastasis of cutaneous melanoma differ between men and women. PLoS One. 2012;7(3):e32955. https://doi.org/10.1371/journal.pone.0032955. PubMed PMID: 22412958; PubMed Central PMCID: PMC3295777.

Nagtegaal ID, Knijn N, Hugen N, Marshall HC, Sugihara K, Tot T, Ueno H, Quirke P. Tumor deposits in colorectal cancer: improving the value of modern staging-a systematic review and meta-analysis. J Clin Oncol. 2017;35(10):1119–27. https://doi.org/10.1200/JCO.2016.68.9091. PubMed PMID: 28029327.

Ratto C, Ricci R, Rossi C, Morelli U, Vecchio FM, Doglietto GB. Mesorectal microfoci adversely affect the prognosis of patients with rectal cancer. Dis Colon Rectum. 2002;45(6):733–42. Discussion 742–3. PubMed PMID: 12072622.

Rock JB, Washington MK, Adsay NV, Greenson JK, Montgomery EA, Robert ME, Yantiss RK, Lehman AM, Frankel WL. Debating deposits: an interobserver variability study of lymph nodes and pericolonic tumor deposits in colonic adenocarcinoma. Arch Pathol Lab Med. 2014;138(5):636–42. https://doi.org/10.5858/arpa.2013-0166-OA. PubMed PMID: 23902577; PubMed Central PMCID:PMC3935980.

Sarioglu S, Akbulut N, Iplikci S, Aydin B, Dogan E, Unlu M, Ellidokuz H, Ada E, Akman F, Ikiz AO. Tumor deposits in head and neck carcinomas. Head Neck. 2016a;38(Suppl 1):E256–60. https://doi.org/10.1002/hed.23981. PubMed PMID: 25546631.

Sarioglu S, Dogan E, Sahin Y, Uzun E, Bekis R, Ada E, Sagol O, Akman F. Undifferentiated laryngeal carcinoma with pagetoid spread. Head Neck Pathol. 2016b;10(2):252–5. https://doi.org/10.1007/s12105-015-0648-7. PubMed PMID: 26292650; PubMed Central PMCID: PMC4838975.

Sobin LH, Gospodarowicz MK, Wittekind CH, editors. International Union against cancer. TNM classification of malignant tumours. 7th ed. West Sussex, England: Wiley-Blackwell; 2009.

Sun Z, Wang ZN, Xu YY, Zhu GL, Huang BJ, Xu Y, Liu FN, Zhu Z, Xu HM. Prognostic significance of tumor deposits in gastric cancer patients who underwent radical surgery. Surgery. 2012;151(6):871–81. https://doi.org/10.1016/j.surg.2011.12.027. PubMed PMID: 22386276.

Ueno H, Mochizuki H, Tamakuma S. Prognostic significance of extranodal microscopic foci discontinuous with primary lesion in rectal cancer. Dis Colon Rectum. 1998;41(1):55–61. PubMed PMID: 9510311.

Ueno H, Mochizuki H, Shirouzu K, Kusumi T, Yamada K, Ikegami M, Kawachi H, Kameoka S, Ohkura Y, Masaki T, Kushima R, Takahashi K, Ajioka Y, Hase K, Ochiai A, Wada R, Iwaya K, Nakamura T, Sugihara K. Study group for tumor deposits without lymph node structure in colorectal cancer projected by the Japanese Society for cancer of the colon and rectum. Multicenter study for optimal categorization of extramural tumor deposits for colorectal cancer staging. Ann Surg. 2012;255(4):739–46. https://doi.org/10.1097/SLA.0b013e31824b4839. PubMed PMID: 22395093.

Wilmott J, Haydu L, Bagot M, Zhang Y, Jakrot V, McCarthy S, Lugassy C, Thompson J, Scolyer R, Barnhill R. Angiotropism is an independent predictor of microscopic satellites in primary cutaneous melanoma. Histopathology. 2012;61(5):889–98. https://doi.org/10.1111/j.1365-2559.2012.04279.x. PubMed PMID: 22716270.

Zhou ZH, Xu GF, Zhang WJ, Zhao HB, Wu YY. Reevaluating significance of perineural invasion in gastric cancer based on double immunohistochemical staining. Arch Pathol Lab Med. 2014;138(2):229–34. https://doi.org/10.5858/arpa.2012-0669-OA. PubMed PMID: 24476520.

Tumor Deposits in Colorectal Cancer

3

Colorectal carcinomas are among the most frequent malignancies of men and women with poor prognosis leading to death. It is the third most common cancer in men and the second in women. More than half of the cases arise in developed countries; however, more than half of the deaths are from the less-developed countries. The variability of the incidence changes tenfold worldwide; however, the sex distribution is less variable considering tumor-related death; women/men is 2/3 (globocan.iarc.fr). The incidence of the colorectal carcinomas decreased during the last decades in patients who are older than 50 but increased in patients younger than that, which may be related to colonoscopy screening for early detection of the cases (Siegel et al. 2017). The progression of carcinoma takes 10–20 years, and median age at diagnosis is 68 years (seer.cancer.gov).

All these data highlight the importance of colorectal carcinoma as a major health problem worldwide.

Prognostic Factors in Colorectal Carcinomas

Mechanisms of colorectal carcinoma progression include more than one molecular pathway. Adenoma carcinoma sequence is by far the most frequent and the one that was recognized earlier. There are two types of genomic instability in colorectal carcinomas: chromosomal instability (CIN), frequently associated with mutated adenomatous polyposis coli gene, and microsatellite instability (MSI), due to DNA repair gene defects. The familial inherited syndromes associated with these two mechanisms are familial polyposis coli syndrome and Lynch syndrome. CpG island mutator phenotype results in silencing of many genes including tumor suppressor genes and or DNA repair genes, resulting in one of the most important mechanisms of colorectal cancer progression. The Consensus Molecular Subtypes (CMS)

S. Sarioglu, *Tumor Deposits*, https://doi.org/10.1007/978-3-319-68582-3_3

Consortium for colorectal carcinomas proposed the following groups considering the accumulating evidence:

- CMS1: MSI immune (14%): Hypermutated, defective mismatch repair, microsatellite instability, MLH-1 silencing, CPH island methylation (CIMP)-high, *BRAF* mutation (+), immune infiltration
- CMS2 (canonical) (37%): Somatic copy number alteration (SCNA) high, *WNT* and *MYC* activation
- CMS3 (metabolic) (13%): SCNA low, CIMP low, *KRAS* mutation, metabolic deregulation, epithelial signature
- CMS4 (mesenchymal) (23%): SCNA high, stromal infiltration, *TGFβ* activation, epithelial-mesenchymal transition, complement activation signature, matrix remodeling
- Mixed features (13%): Transition phenotype, intratumoral heterogeneity (Müller et al. 2016; Arends 2013)

The morphological types of carcinomas also have prognostic value. The most common types of colorectal carcinomas are low- and high-grade adenocarcinomas (Fig. 3.1). The poor prognostic types are signet-ring cell (Fig. 3.2) and high-grade neuroendocrine carcinoma. Mucinous, signet-ring, medullary, serrated, and large-cell neuroendocrine carcinoma and adenosquamous, mixed adenoneuroendocrine, squamous cell, micropapillary, spindle cell, and undifferentiated carcinoma are the other types (Figures 3.3, 3.4, 3.5, 3.6, 3.7, 3.8, and 3.9). Our colorectal oncology group, as well as many other researchers, has evaluated angiogenesis, lymphatic and vascular invasion, desmoplasia, adhesion molecule expressions, matrix metalloproteinases, tumor suppressor genes, and markers of hypoxia, as markers of prognosis in colorectal carcinomas (Sokmen et al. 2001a, Sokmen et al. 2001b, Cooper et al. 2003, Sis et al 2005, Lebe et al 2005, Tuna et al 2006, Cavdar et al 2009, Arslan et al 2014); however, none of these factors provided strong evidence to be included in TNM classification which provide the most important prognostic information. Perineural, lymphatic, and vascular invasion and tubular and circumferential margins are included in the prognostic factors that are valuable enough to be included in CAP templates for colorectal carcinomas (CAP). Tumor budding provided strong evidence as a poor prognostic factor, with increased risk of lymph node metastasis, tumor recurrence, as well as tumor-related death, more than four times; however, it is included in neither CAP protocol nor TNM classification (Ueno et al. 2002; Rogers et al. 2016). One of the most important prognostic factors included in both guidelines is tumor deposits and will be further discussed in detail.

Proposed Mechanisms and Morphology of TDs in Colorectal Carcinomas

TDs have been named as tumor nodule, microfoci, neoplastic foci, tumor aggregate, extrabowel skipped cancer infiltration, discontinuous carcinoma, extranodal foci, non-nodal metastatic foci, extranodal cancer deposits, and isolated tumor deposits in the literature (Nagtegaal and Quirke 2007).

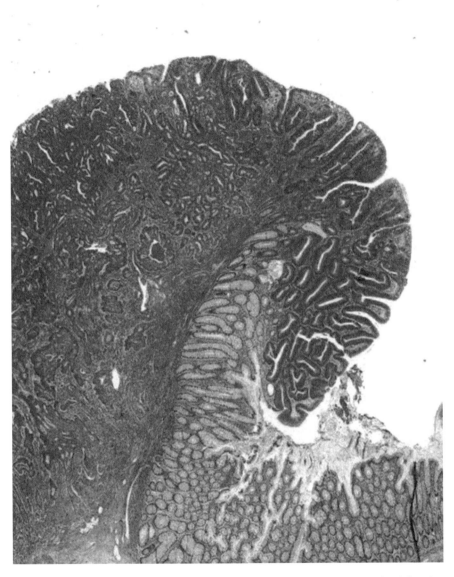

Fig. 3.1 Low-grade adenocarcinoma arising from an adenoma (Normal mucosa at the *right*, tubular adenoma at the middle and adenocarcinoma at the *left*). The most common form of colorectal carcinoma and the morphological evidence of the progression from adenoma. The sequence of molecular events in this case is nicely described, including adenomatous polyposis coli (APC), *KRAS*, deleted in colorectal cancer (*DCC*), and *p53* mutations in a stepwise fashion) (H&E original magnification ×10)

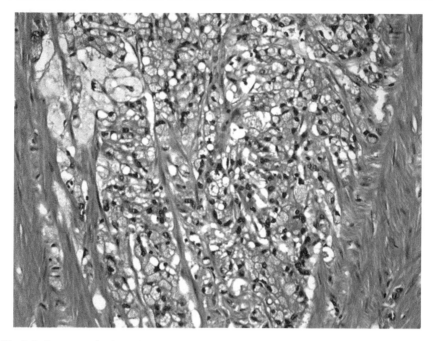

Fig. 3.2 Rare type of colorectal carcinoma made up of signet-ring cells rich in intracellular mucin (H&E original magnification ×40)

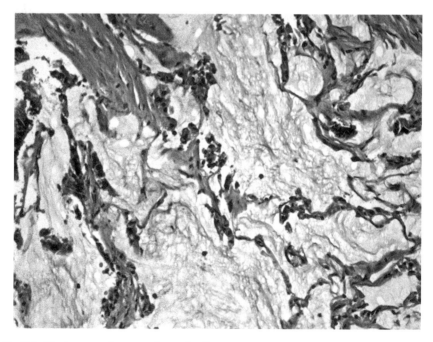

Fig. 3.3 Mucinous carcinoma made up of malignant tumor cells swimming in mucin pools (H&E original magnification ×20)

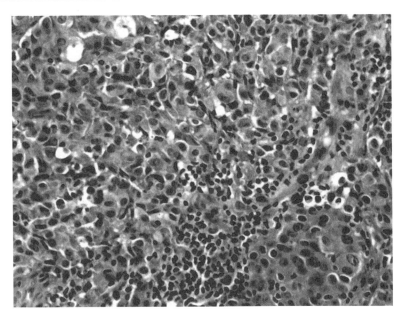

Fig. 3.4 Medullary carcinoma. The tumor was located at the cecum; many lymphocytes were infiltrating the malignant cells with large cytoplasm. There was loss of *PMS2* and *MLH1* expression, with high microsatellite instability (*BAT-25*, *BAT-26*, *D2S123*, *D5S346*, and *D17S250* were unstable). Medullary carcinoma is a rare tumor that may be associated with Lynch syndrome (H&E original magnification ×40)

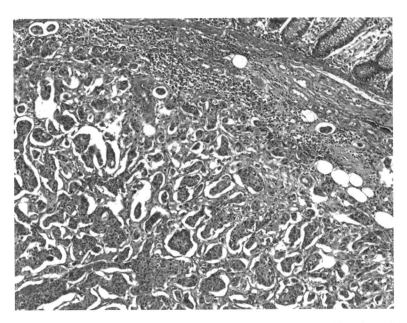

Fig. 3.5 Micropapillary pattern was first described in breast carcinomas, and later it was identified in tumors from different organs including colorectal carcinomas, and it is suggested that this type of tumor forming small tumor clusters without a vascular structure and stroma share some similarities with tumor buds. More frequent lymphatic invasion, lymph node metastasis, and poor prognosis seem to be associated with these tumors (H&E original magnification ×20)

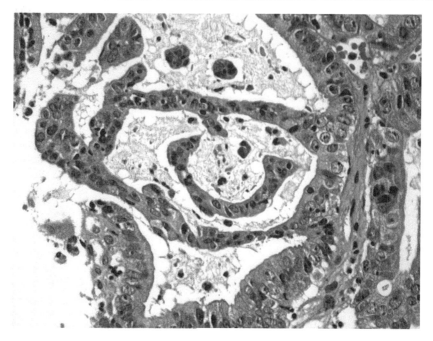

Fig. 3.6 Serrated adenocarcinoma with large cytoplasm, vesicular nuclei, and rod-shaped free structures; mucinous areas may also be observed. This type of tumors is associated with serrated adenomas/polyps, CIMP-positive status, *BRAF* mutations, and relatively better survival; MSI is rare (H&E original magnification ×20)

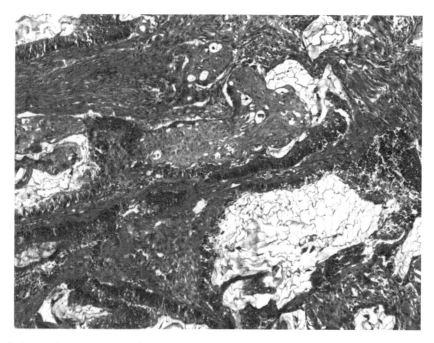

Fig. 3.7 Adenosquamous carcinoma, a rare tumor with dual differentiation (H&E original magnification ×20)

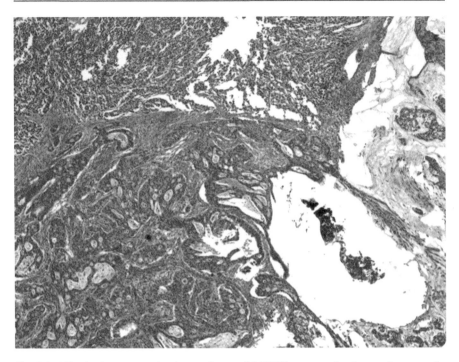

Fig. 3.8 Mixed adenoneuroendocrine carcinoma (MANEC); neuroendocrine carcinoma at the upper part and adenocarcinoma at the inferior region (H&E original magnification ×10)

TDs are discontinuous neoplastic masses from the primary tumor at the lymphatic draining area. They probably represent extensive extramural venous or perineural invasion as in most cases the TDs are associated with these structures. There has been a 3 mm cut point for naming a lesion as TD; however, there is no strict evidence that these lesions are different from a lesion that has a smaller diameter. In the series of colon carcinomas, Goldstein and Turner (2000) found that TD with any diameter was a poor prognostic factor for disease-free survival. Finding very tiny lesions during macroscopic examination would be unreliable if the lesions were not submitted in toto for microscopic examination. However, the frequent desmoplastic reaction surrounding the TD may allow easier palpation for pathologists during macroscopic examination.

There is not much study comparing the molecular mechanisms of lymph node metastasis and TDs. In a series of 193 colorectal carcinomas, the epithelial-mesenchymal transition markers, Twist and Snail expressions, as well as their target which is repressed by them, E-cadherin expression, were evaluated. Snail expression was significantly more frequent in cases with lymph node metastasis, while Twist expression was more frequent in cases with TDs. Snail was identified as a predictor of lymph node metastasis, and Twist was a predictor of TD formation. The authors suggested that different mechanisms operated during these two processes, metastasis to lymph nodes and TD formation. The expressions of Twist and Snail were also predictors of metastasis (Fan et al. 2013).

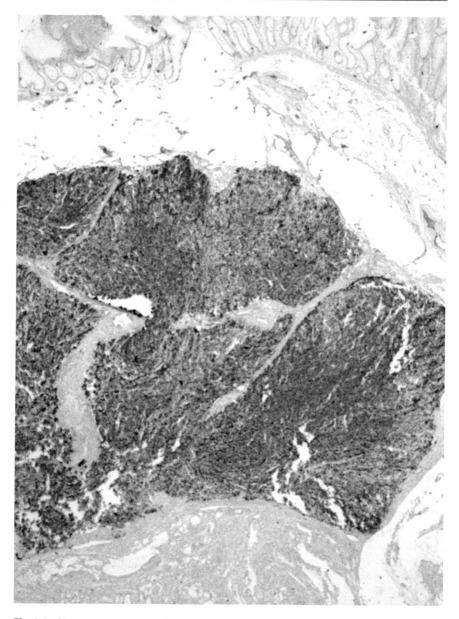

Fig. 3.9 Chromogranin-A expression at the neuroendocrine component and negative results at the adenocarcinoma region at the lower part (same case Fig. 3.8) (IHC original magnification ×5)

The diagnosis of a metastatic lymph node or a TD may be straightforward in many cases, but in some lesions it is challenging to choose one of these categories. However the morphology of the lesions which may be included among TDs may present some differences. Some of these raise diagnostic challenges like if the lesion is a TD or a metastatic lymph node. Morphological subtypes of tumor deposits, which will be discussed in the following sections may cause different diagnostic challenges. There are a few interobserver agreement studies. In a series by Ueno et al. (2012), 109 randomly selected extramural lesions were evaluated by 11 observers from 11 institutions. The κ value for lymph node metastasis and TD was 0.74; for vascular invasion type and irregular contour type, it was 0.63; and for perineural type and irregular contour type, it was 0.64. The κ values for smooth contour type with the other types were the lowest (0.51). A group of gastrointestinal pathologists selected 25 challenging lesions and evaluated their interobserver agreement and features that were valuable in diagnosis. Complete agreement was achieved in 11 (44%) cases: five metastatic lymph nodes and six tumor deposits; however, there was disagreement in more than half of the cases, and κ statistic was 0.48 (Rock et al. 2014). The authors expressed that the most helpful morphological features during the evaluation of the lesions to reach a diagnosis included round shape, lymphocytic rim, subcapsular sinus, residual lymph node, and a thick capsule. In these cases, elastin stains were not helpful in any of the cases, but serial sections were helpful in three (12%) cases. The authors noted that lymphoid follicles and lymphoid rim are features of carcinomas with microsatellite instability and should not be a reliable feature for a diagnosis of metastatic lymph node. The results highlight the difficulties in the diagnosis of extramural lesions as metastatic lymph nodes and tumor deposits, at least in a group of the lesions, even among the experts in the field of gastrointestinal pathology.

Classifications of TDs in Colorectal Carcinomas

TDs were first identified in colorectal carcinomas as early as 1935 by Gabriel et al. (1935). The morphological differences between TDs seem to be related to differences of their pathogenesis. In order to understand the pathogenesis, morphology, and prognostic importance of TDs, different features of these lesions were evaluated which may be listed as follows:

– Size
– Contour
– Number
– Patterns like scattering, perivascular, perineural, and nodular
– Morphological relation with vascular, lymphatic, and neural structures (Goldstein and Turner 2000)

In different series, different classifications of TD were used. This results in difficulties of comparison between different series.

In the study by Ueno et al. (2007), the TDs were named as extranodal cancer deposits (EX), and they were classified into morphological categories reflecting the possible morphological variants as follows:

– Vascular invasion type: Deposits adjacent to vascular structures
– Nonvascular: Deposits that are not adjacent to vascular or neural structures
– Aggressive EX: Nonvascular invasion-type EX following active venous or neural invasion

Shimada and Takii (2010) classified the EX as follows:

- EX invading lymphatic vessels, veins, or perineural tissue
- EX with smooth contours
- EX with irregular contours

In a multicenter study by Ueno et al. (2012), the extramural lesions were classified as follows:

- Cancer foci mostly confined to the vascular or perineural spaces (vascular invasion/neural invasion, VAS/NI)
- Smooth contoured tumor nodule (S-ND)
- Irregularly contoured tumor nodule (I-ND)

Goldstein and Turner (2000) reviewed the images and classifications in older literature and compared them with the ones they named as TDs. They stated that the lesions that they named as TDs in their study were classified as extramural spread, foci of perineural invasion, extramural venous invasion, or lymph nodes replaced by the neoplastic cells.

Tumor staging depending upon tumor, node, and distant metastasis was proposed in 1940 by Pierre Denoix, a French surgeon (Greene 2012), and this has been used increasingly, and for many decades, it has been the most important prognostic factor in nearly all solid tumors. The importance of TDs in colorectal carcinomas was striking, and they were included in TNM classifications since 1997. However, their role has not been settled yet. They were categorized in T or N and even M categories during the last two decades (Table 3.1).

Table 3.1 The classifications of the extramural tumor deposits in AJCC classifications 1997, 2002, 2007, and 2017 (Sobin LH et al. 1997, Sobin LH et al. 2002, Sobin LH et al. 2010, Brierley J et al. 2017)

Year		Classification
1997	TNM5	Pericolonic tumor deposits more than 3 mm should be classified as a metastatic lymph node; if less than 3 mm, these are accepted as discontinuous adenocarcinoma (pT3)
2002	TNM6	Pericolonic tumor deposits with smooth contours should be classified as a metastatic lymph node; if the contours are not smooth, then the deposit should be named as vascular invasion
2010	TNM7	All the cases with TD but without lymph node metastasis should be classified as N1c; these lesions should not be classified in T category. If the tumor nodule has smooth contours with morphological evidence allowing to be named as a lymph node extensively invaded by carcinoma, then it should be counted as a metastatic lymph node
2017	TNM8	Tumor deposits should not have histological evidence of residual lymph node or identifiable vascular or neural structures. If a vessel wall is identifiable on H&E or other stains, it should be classified as either venous (V1/2) or lymphatic invasion (L1). If neural structures are identifiable, the lesion should be classified as perineural invasion (Pn1). Tumor deposits do not change the primary tumor T category, but change the node status (N) to N1c if all regional lymph nodes are negative on pathological examination

The 1997 TNM *AJCC Cancer Staging Handbook* (AJCC98), the 5th edition, stated that tumor deposit in pericolonic adipose tissue should be classified as a metastatic lymph node in case its diameter was more than 3 mm. If the deposit was less than 3 mm diameter, it was considered as discontinuous adenocarcinoma at least pT3 (TNM AJCC 1997). At the 6th edition at 2002, it was stated that a deposit with smooth contours should be classified as a metastatic lymph node even if there was no structural evidence of a lymph node. In case the contours are irregular, the deposit should be named as venous invasion, either V1 if it may be only detected with microscopic examination or V2 if it is evident that the tumor has macroscopical perivascular invasion (TNM AJCC 2002).

According to their findings, in 2007, Ueno et al. suggested that the best prognostic information was achieved if the TDs were grouped as lymph nodes, changing the N stage, excluding the vascular invasion type of TD which should be accepted as tumor growth, and if this was observed, only T stage might change.

In 2009, Puppa et al. suggested that for the TNM staging system of colorectal cancer, a method similar to melanoma should be applied as the perivascular and perineural disseminations of TDs are similar to the melanoma in-transit metastasis. TDs without a lymph node structure and that are associated with nerves or vessels should be considered as M1a category as well as aggressive TDs (scattering pattern, not surrounded by lymphocytes). The cases with distant (visceral) metastases should be designated to the M1b category.

Belt et al. (2010) reported the poor prognosis of colorectal carcinomas cases with TD and suggested that any stage II case with TD should be classified in stage III category. At the same year, 2010, at the 7th edition of the UICC classification, pN1c category was introduced for the cases without lymph node metastasis but positive for TD/TDs. If the deposit has smooth contours persuading the pathologist that it once had been a lymph node, then it should be classified as a metastatic lymph node (Sobin et al. 2009, Edge SB et al. 2010).

In 2011 Nagtegaal ID et al. evaluated a series of 960 cases from two centers according to the 5th, 6th, and 7th editions of TNM classification. The reproducibility of TNM5 was better than TNM6. They reported N and T stage changes with changes in the classification causing upstaging and downstaging. According to TNM5, 6, and 7, 34.4, 38.2, and 43.1% of the patients were classified as stage III, respectively, and would or would not receive chemotherapy accordingly. If stage II cases with high-risk features were included, the percentage of the cases turned out to be 57.8, 64.1, and 64.7, respectively, with different staging schemes. N changes were more frequent than T category. These discrepancies of stages result in many important problems like:

- Changing treatment modalities
- Confusing old histopathology reports
- Difficulties in prognostic studies
- Loss of interobserver reliability due to changing and non-detailed criteria for TD

Qiu et al. (2011) applied Akaike information criterion in a series of colorectal cancer cases which were evaluated for TD and prognosis; their results were also like the findings of Ueno et al. in 2007, in which when cases of TDs were classified as metastatic lymph nodes, best information was achieved.

Al Sahaf et al. (2011) suggested that the TDs should be included in the M category due to the poor prognosis of the cases compatible with stage IV disease.

In a multicenter study by 11 observers, TDs were evaluated by including them in T and N categories and found that stronger prognostic value was achieved if they were included in N category and this would overcome the problems with interobserver reliability. If they were excluded from both T and N categories, worst prognostic information was achieved. They noted that as the number of T1 and T2 cases was very small in their series, they could not conclude about the T stage and extramural vascular or perineural deposits, and further evaluation was required in larger series. Song et al. (2012) found similar results in a series of 513 colorectal carcinoma cases. Contrary to these findings in a series by Yabata et al. (2014) including colorectal carcinoma cases, the only independent prognostic factor was TDs with a hazard ratio of 2.813. Recurrences were observed in 49.2% of the patients with TDs and 14.4% of the patients who did not have TDs. Yabata et al. suggested that the prognostic impact of TDs was between lymph node and distant metastasis.

In a series by Jin et al. (2015) of 438 right-sided colon adenocarcinoma cases, pN1c cases were compared with other N categories, and they concluded that metastatic lymph nodes and TDs had similar impact on prognosis.

The latest 2017 TNM classification, the 8th edition, changed the classifications once again. This time the existence of tumor deposits were accepted only if there was no lymph node metastasis and named as pN1c, only if they were not associated with residual lymph nodes and vascular and neural structures. If there was a metastatic lymph node, the TDs are counted as metastatic lymph nodes. If a vessel wall or neural structure is identified, then the lesion should be named as venous invasion or perineural invasion.

This list of proposals and changes of classification reflects that the issues have not been solved yet.

Prognostic Studies on Tumor Deposits in Colorectal Carcinomas

Some of the prognostic information from multiple studies about tumor deposits in colorectal carcinomas is summarized under the "Classifications of TDs in Colorectal Carcinomas" heading, in order to discuss the mechanisms for proposals for classification. In this section, this information is detailed further.

TDs were recognized as poor prognostic factors in colorectal adenocarcinomas. In the series of Goldstein and Turner (2000), 400 pT3 cases with lymph node metastasis but without distant metastasis were evaluated for the prognostic value of TDs, in terms of disease-free survival. In this series, 18% of the cases had TDs and measured 1–10.2 mm. The TDs were associated with the number of metastatic lymph nodes, increasing tumor grade, as well as extramural venous invasion. When cases were stratified as none, 1 or 2 TDs, and 3 or more TDs, the actuarial 5-year survival rates were 35%, 24%, and 2%, respectively. In the multivariate analysis, number of metastatic lymph nodes, tumor grade and TDs were independent factors, for metastatic diseases and increased the risk of metastatic disease 1.5 times. In a second model, the number of TDs was included and identified as an independent prognostic factor with a risk ratio of 1.05. For the cases with TDs, the maximum dimension of TDs was identified as an independent prognostic factor as well as the number of metastatic lymph nodes and tumor grade with a risk ratio of 1.95. In cases with TDs, the rate of intra-abdominal metastasis was significantly higher related to both the number and diameter of the TDs. Furthermore, for any TD with any diameter, including the ones smaller than 3 mm were associated with shorter disease-free survival.

Intra-abdominal metastasis was more frequent and earlier in cases with TDs. An increased number of TDs increased the intra-abdominal metastasis with an odds ratio of 5.3. Two hundred and seven patients developed metastatic disease. Of these, in the ones without TDs, 12% had intra-abdominal metastases and 47% had hepatic metastasis, while in cases with TDs, 59% had intra-abdominal metastasis and 24% had hepatic metastasis as the initial metastatic sites. In 30 cases, the TDs were evaluated by step sections in order to identify their origins, and more than 70% of the cases were associated with perineural, perivascular, and intravascular growth and in some cases a combination of these. All the cases were associated with at least one of these.

In the series of Ueno et al. (2007), of 1027 cases of colorectal carcinomas, 20% of the cases had EX. EX were more frequent in rectal carcinoma cases (23.3%) compared with colon cases (16.6%). Aggressive type of EX was rare and was identified in 6.8% of cases but had a hazard ratio of 8.0 in univariate analysis. They identified EX diameter as a poor prognostic factor especially for cases with deposits larger than 10 mm. Nonvascular type was more frequent; the hazard ratios for cases with metastatic lymph nodes, vascular type, and nonvascular types were 3.6, 2.5, and 4.7, respectively. Multivariate analysis was carried out only in these three groups, and only lymph node metastasis and nonvascular EX were found as poor prognostic factors.

In the series by Shimada and Takii (2010), whole tissues of the specimens were evaluated with microscopic sections from 214 stage I–III rectal carcinoma cases, and TDs were identified in 41.1% of the series. In the multivariate analysis, the hazard ratios for the independent prognostic factors, which included only metastatic lymph nodes and EX, are 2.1 and 7.6, respectively. When types of TDs were considered, the independent prognostic factors for disease-free survival were metastatic lymph nodes, vascular/perineural invasion-type TDs, smooth nodule-type TDs, and irregular nodule-type TDs, and the hazard ratios were 4.1, 4.2, 4.7, and 5.6, respectively. The independent prognostic factors for overall survival included tumor size (the cut point was 40 mm), nodal involvement, and EX with hazard ratios of 2.7, 2.4 and 6.7, respectively. This study presented a very detailed method for finding the EX, and none of the patients had received neoadjuvant therapy. The higher percentage of EX in this series probably reflects the real incidence of TD in rectal carcinoma as they may be missed during macroscopic examination; in this case, whole-mount sections are more reliable. They identified EX as a worse prognostic factor compared with nodal metastasis.

In the series of Belt et al. (2010), of 870 cases of colorectal carcinomas, some of which received neoadjuvant therapy, TDs were observed in 14.8% of the cases and more frequent in cases with lymph node metastasis (8.2 vs. 25.3%). In stage II TD (+) and (−) cases, tumor recurrence was observed in 50 vs. 24.4% of the cases, and TD was identified as an independent prognostic factor as in many series.

Qiu et al. (2011) evaluated TD in 1215 patients with colorectal cancer. TDs were found in 13.7% of the patients. TDs, pN, tumor size, differentiation, and pT were independent prognostic factors in multivariate analysis.

Al Sahaf et al. (2011) evaluated perinodal invasion as well as TD in stage II and III colon carcinomas as prognostic markers. They found lymph node ratio, extracapsular lymph node extension, and adjuvant chemotherapy as independent prognostic markers of both disease-free survival and overall survival (odds ratios of 2.2, 3.0, and 0.56 and 2.6, 1.95, and 0.235, respectively), and TDs were important for overall survival (odds ratio of 1.77). TD was associated with an 11% 5-year survival rate, and perinodal invasion was associated with a 33% 5-year survival rate.

In a series by Yabata et al. (2014), including colorectal carcinoma cases who did not receive neoadjuvant therapy, considering the cases with lymph node metastasis, the only prognostic factor identified with Cox model, among age, positive radial surgical margin, tumor depth, TDs, lymphatic invasion, and venous invasion, was TDs with a hazard ratio of 2.813. Recurrences were observed in 49.2% of the patients with TDs and 14.4% of the patients who did not have TDs. This study presents that when TDs are accepted as metastatic lymph nodes, the importance of TDs which are associated with worse prognosis is overlooked among the cases with lymph node metastasis. Yabata et al. suggested that the prognostic impact of TDs was between lymph node and distant metastasis.

In the series of 513 colorectal carcinoma cases by Song et al. (2012), the TDs were counted as lymph nodes, and this resulted in N stage migration of patients in 88 (58%) cases out of 151 patients with TDs. They found better results for predicting prognosis when TDs were classified among metastatic lymph nodes; furthermore, the prognosis of patients at the same pN stages was not different whether TDs were added or not and concluded that the impact of a TD is as strong as metastatic lymph node.

In a series by Jin et al. (2015) of 438 right-sided colon adenocarcinoma cases, the cases classified as pN1c according to TNM 2010 classification were compared with pN0, pN1, and pN2 cases. pN1c cases had worse prognosis than pN0 and better prognosis than pN2 cases. While statistically insignificant, they had poorer prognosis than pN1 cases. pN1 cases ($N = 17$) were further subdivided into cases with <4 or ≥4 TDs, and the group with more TDs had significantly worse prognosis (median survival time of 32.5 and 16.5 months, respectively). They concluded that the impact of TDs was similar to metastatic lymph nodes.

In a series of 385 M0, T3–T4 cases of colorectal carcinoma cases by Yamano et al. (2015), TDs were evaluated and grouped as smooth and irregularly contoured. Extranodal invasion was an independent prognostic factor for colon carcinoma cases for relapse-free survival, and smooth and irregularly contoured TDs or all contours were significant prognostic factors for relapse-free survival, and irregularly contoured TDs were significant for disease-specific survival. They concluded that extranodal invasion and TDs provide valuable prognostic information for colorectal carcinoma patients.

Discussion About TDs in Colorectal Carcinomas

Many studies presented the poor prognostic influence of TDs in colorectal carcinomas. Diagnosis of TDs is very important for patient management in colorectal carcinomas and neglecting the identification of the lesions properly is of utmost importance. However, for many lesions, the typing is a difficult issue.

Some example images are presented:

Figure 3.10: Tumor 2 mm away from the muscularis propria, a little bigger than 3 mm and adjacent to vascular structures. The last classification TNM8 seems to include this lesion as venous invasion, but we cannot see any vascular invasion as in many cases giving pathologists a hard time in making a diagnosis that one does not observe. Considering the regular contours, this lesion is not also an excellent example for vascular invasion which is generally described in association with irregular contours.

Figure 3.11: Small tumor foci surrounding peripheral nerves. This is a lesion that may be easily diagnosed as perineural invasion.

Figure 3.12: In this case, the tumor cells make a small cluster surrounding the blood vessels, and the lesion is a typical example of extramural perivascular migratory invasion, which is not a terminology associated with adenocarcinomas but one that is used in malignant melanomas.

Figure 3.13: At the serial sections of the previous case, the extramural perivascular migratory invasion expanded resulting in a tumor mass larger than 3 mm. In this case, according to the latest TNM classification, this lesion is named as vascular invasion, but morphologically there is no vascular invasion.

Figure 3.14: A large TD with irregular contours; adenocarcinoma and squamous cell carcinoma morphologies are intermingled. Vascular or neural structures cannot be identified, and no residual lymph node structures are observed. This lesion is in the TD category in any of the classifications.

Figure 3.15: A tiny tumoral lesion, which is not adjacent to a vascular structure and without evidence of lymph node structures. This lesion was smaller than 3 mm even in serial sections.

Figure 3.16: Three lesions are seen adjacent to each other. The one at the right and middle should be named as vascular invasion, but one of them was a TD at the previous classification. The one at the right seems to be a TD if the lesion is devoid of vascular, neural, and lymph node structures in serial sections.

Figure 3.17: Tumor with smooth contours lacking lymph node structures, adjacent to vascular structures. It is hard to determine if this is a tumor deposit with smooth contours or a metastatic lymph node. Furthermore, as there are vascular structures at the right side, this lesion may even be classified as vascular invasion.

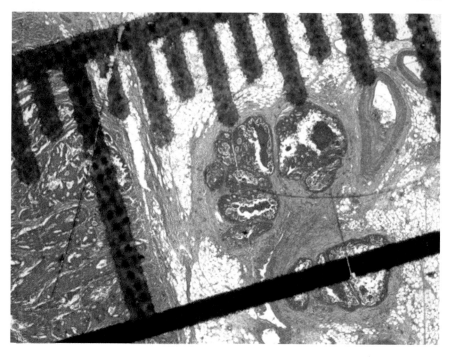

Fig. 3.10   Example from a colorectal carcinoma case (H&E original magnification ×10)

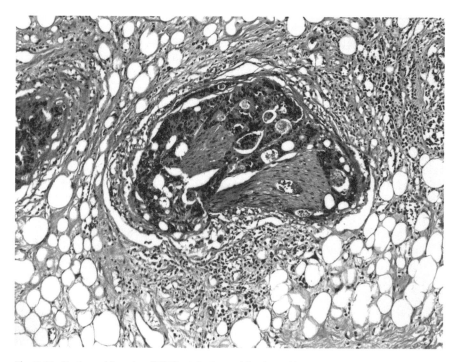

Fig. 3.11   Perineural invasion (H&E original magnification ×40)

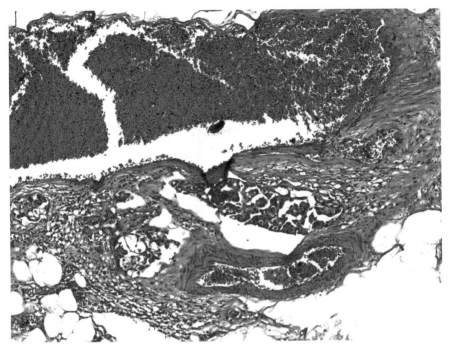

Fig. 3.12 Extramural perivascular invasion (H&E original magnification ×20)

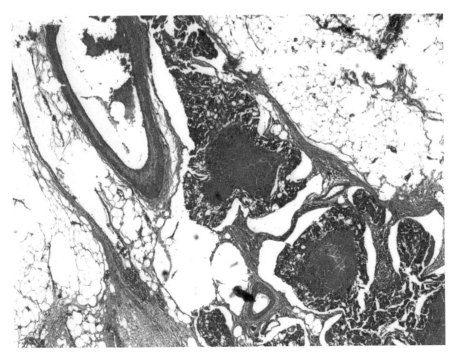

Fig. 3.13 Extramural tumor mass (H&E original magnification ×20)

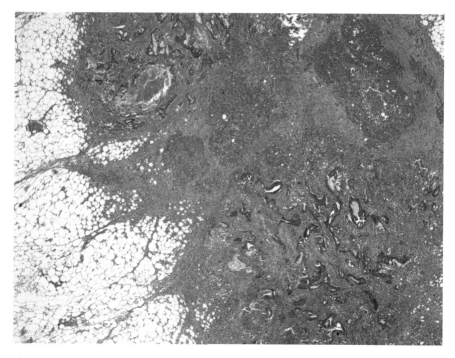

Fig. 3.14 A TD arising from an adenosquamous carcinoma (H&E original magnification ×5)

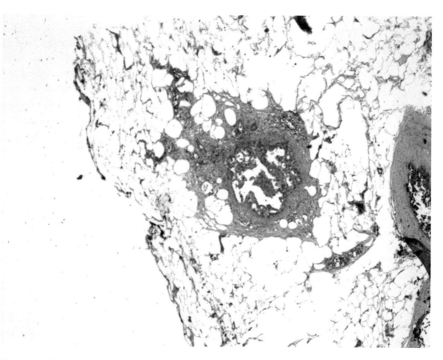

Fig. 3.15 Tiny lesion less than 3 mm (H&E original magnification ×5)

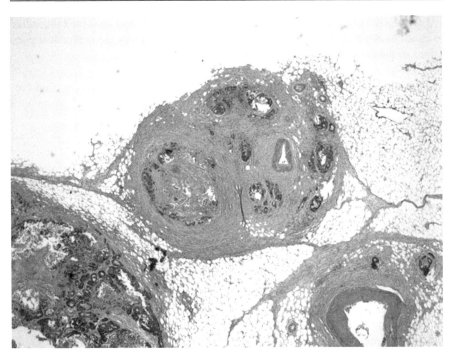

Fig. 3.16 Multiple lesions with different morphological features (H&E original magnification ×5)

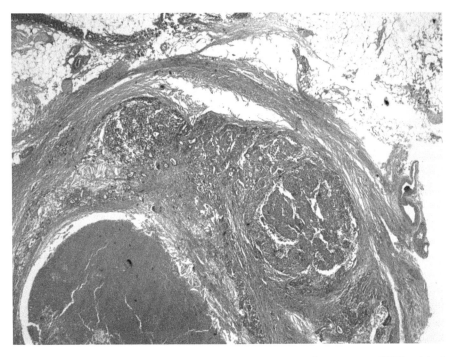

Fig. 3.17 Smooth contoured malignant lesion adjacent to vascular structures (H&E original magnification ×5)

During the evaluation of the cases, multiple challenges may be solved if the classifications depend upon morphological evidence. At this part the personal suggestions of the author are presented:

- Lesions with smooth contours should be accepted as tumor deposits if no lymphoid sinuses are observed. Lymphocytes, lymphoid follicles, and peritumoral fibrosis are not specific for lymph nodes.
- Lesions adjacent to lymphatics, peripheral nerves, and blood vessels but not actually invading the structures like in Figs. 3.12, 3.13, and 3.14 should be named as tumor deposits. The lesions in 12 should be named as "extravascular migratory metastasis of perineural type," and lesions in 13 and 14 should be named as "extravascular migratory metastasis of vascular type."
- Diagnosis of "vascular invasion" should be spared only for cases with intravascular tumor cells attached to the endothelial layer covered by fibrin thrombi.
- Extravascular migratory metastasis of vascular type should be accepted as one of the basic pathways of dissemination in addition to lymphatic vascular and perineural invasion.
- In cases with either TDs or metastatic lymph nodes receiving chemotherapy, an increased number of metastatic lymph nodes and TDs are associated with poor prognosis, and the pathology reports should include the number of metastatic lymph nodes and the number of TDs, but the N stage should be given according to the sum of both, and N stage should be named as combined N stage.

Neoadjuvant Radiotherapy and Tumor Deposits

Neoadjuvant treatment of rectal carcinoma has decreased the local recurrences, and it is the standard of care in many countries. The histopathological evaluation of the radical surgery specimens of such cases following this type of therapy raises many questions including:

- What is the meaning of mucin pools at the intestinal wall and in the lymph nodes?
- If a tumor is not identified macroscopically, what type of tissue processing and sectioning should be performed?
- How to understand if the histopathological features like mucinous or neuroendocrine type of differentiation are related to the primary tumor histopathology or post-therapy changes.

– Furthermore, tumor deposits are hard to define in these cases as, with tumor regression, remnants of the tumor may be observed at any size and location. In many series about the tumor deposits in colorectal carcinomas, colon carcinoma cases and rectal carcinoma cases that did not receive neoadjuvant therapy are included and the others are excluded (Hav et al. 2015).

Short-course radiotherapy does not result in downstaging, but long-course adjuvant therapy and waiting 6–12 weeks till surgery change the T and N stage considerably. It is hard to apply TD rules in these cases as residual (micro) tumor foci are observed in 17–48% of these cases (Nagtegaal et al. 2011). However, it is hard to be sure if these are TDs or tumor remnants of T3 cases.

In the series of Ratto et al. (2007), a series of 68 cases which received neoadjuvant radiotherapy were analyzed for metastatic microfoci, and these were found in 38.2% of the cases. They found no TDs in cases with total tumor regression.

Some examples of post-radiotherapy lesions are presented in Figs. 3.18, 3.19, and 3.20; markers for distinction between primary and metastatic tumors either as a metastatic lymph node or TDs are required.

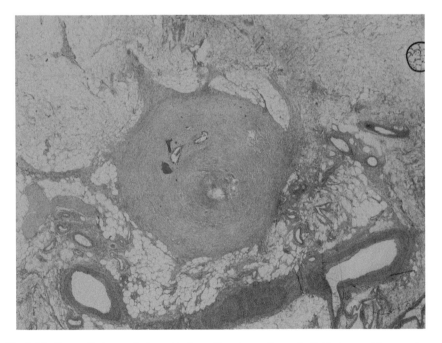

Fig. 3.18 Post-radiotherapy lesion with dense fibrosis; small neoplastic foci are not far away from vascular structures. This may represent a TD (H&E original magnification ×10)

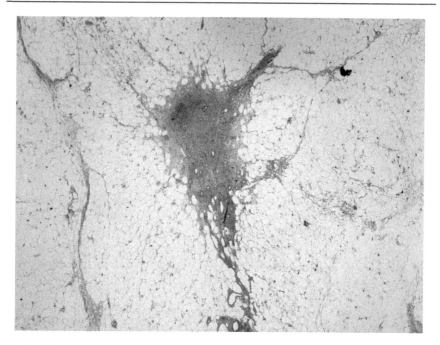

Fig. 3.19 Post-radiotherapy lesion with dense fibrosis and small neoplastic foci. It is hard to be sure if this lesion is a TD or remnant neoplastic tissue with post-radiotherapy changes (H&E original magnification ×5)

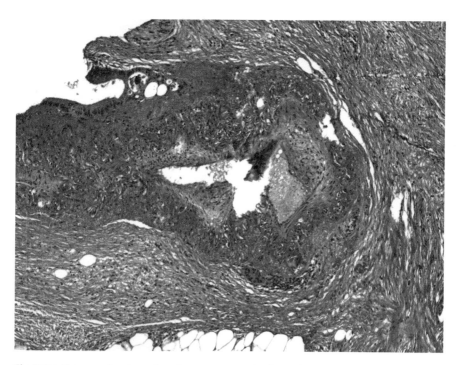

Fig. 3.20 Extramural perivascular migratory metastasis of vascular type may be seen also in post-radiotherapy cases (H&E original magnification ×10)

References

AJCC staging handbook. 6th ed. New York: Springer; 2002.

Al Sahaf O, Myers E, Jawad M, Browne TJ, Winter DC, Redmond HP. The prognostic significance of extramural deposits and extracapsular lymph node invasion in colon cancer. Dis Colon Rectum. 2011;54(8):982–8. https://doi.org/10.1097/DCR.0b013e31821c4944. PubMed PMID: 21730787.

American Joint Committee on Cancer. Purposes and principles of staging. In: Fleming ID, Cooper JS, Henson DE, Hutter RVP, Kennedy BJ, Murphy GP, et al., editors. AJCC cancer staging handbook. 5th ed. Philadelphia: LippincottRaven; 1998. p. 10.

Arends MJ. Pathways of colorectal carcinogenesis. Appl Immunohistochem Mol Morphol. 2013;21(2):97–102. https://doi.org/10.1097/PAI.0b013e31827ea79e. Review. PubMed PMID: 23417071.

Arslan NC, Sokmen S, Canda AE, Terzi C, Sarioglu S. The prognostic impact of the log odds of positive lymph nodes in colon cancer. Color Dis. 2014;16(11):O386–92. https://doi.org/10.1111/codi.12702. PubMed PMID: 24980876.

Belt EJ, van Stijn MF, Bril H, de Lange-de Klerk ES, Meijer GA, Meijer S, Stockmann HB. Lymph node negative colorectal cancers with isolated tumor deposits should be classified and treated as stage III. Ann Surg Oncol. 2010;17(12):3203–11. https://doi.org/10.1245/s10434-010-1152-7. Epub 2010 Jul 13. PubMed PMID: 20625841; PubMed Central PMCID: PMC2995864.

Brierley J, Gospodarowicz M, Wittekind C. UICC TNM classification of malignant tumours. Eighth ed. Chichester: Wiley; 2017.

Cavdar Z, Canda AE, Terzi C, Sarioglu S, Fuzun M, Oktay G. Role of gelatinases (matrix metalloproteinases 2 and 9), vascular endothelial growth factor and endostatin on clinicopathological behaviour of rectal cancer. Color Dis. 2011;13(2):154–60. https://doi.org/10.1111/j.1463-1318.2009.02105.x. PubMed PMID: 19888958.

Cooper R, Sarioğlu S, Sökmen S, Füzün M, Küpelioğlu A, Valentine H, Görken IB, Airley R, West C. Glucose transporter-1 (GLUT-1): a potential marker of prognosis in rectal carcinoma? Br J Cancer. 2003;89(5):870–6. PubMed PMID: 12942120; PubMed Central PMCID: PMC2394489.

Edge SB, Byrd DR, Compton CC, et al. AJCC cancer staging manual. 7th ed. New York: Springer; 2010.

Fan XJ, Wan XB, Yang ZL, Fu XH, Huang Y, Chen DK, Song SX, Liu Q, Xiao HY, Wang L, Wang JP. Snail promotes lymph node metastasis and Twist enhances tumor deposit formation through epithelial-mesenchymal transition in colorectal cancer. Hum Pathol. 2013;44(2):173–80. https://doi.org/10.1016/j.humpath.2012.03.029. Epub 2012 Sep 10. PubMed PMID: 22974478.

Gabriel WB, Dukes CE, Bussey HJR. Lymphatic spread in cancer of the rectum. Br J Surg. 1935;23:395–413.

Goldstein NS, Turner JR. Pericolonic tumor deposits in patients with T3N+MO colon adenocarcinomas: markers of reduced disease free survival and intra-abdominal metastases and their implications for TNM classification. Cancer. 2000;88(10):2228–38. PubMed PMID: 10820343.

Greene FL. Tumor deposits in colorectal cancer: a moving target. Ann Surg. 2012;255(2):214–5. https://doi.org/10.1097/SLA.0b013e3182430eaa. PubMed PMID: 22202583.

Hav M, Libbrecht L, Ferdinande L, Geboes K, Pattyn P, Cuvelier CA. Pathologic assessment of rectal carcinoma after neoadjuvant radio(chemo)therapy: prognostic implications. Biomed Res Int. 2015;2015:574540. https://doi.org/10.1155/2015/574540. Epub 2015 Oct 5. Review. PubMed PMID: 26509160; PubMed Central PMCID: PMC4609786.

http://globocan.iarc.fr/Pages/fact_sheets_cancer.aspx. Accessed Apr 2017.

http://www.cap.org/ShowProperty?nodePath=/UCMCon/Contribution%20Folders/WebContent/pdf/cp-colon-16protocol-3400.pdf. Accessed May 2017.

https://seer.cancer.gov/statfacts/html/colorect.html. Accessed Apr 2017.

Jin M, Roth R, Rock JB, Washington MK, Lehman A, Frankel WL. The impact of tumor deposits on colonic adenocarcinoma AJCC TNM staging and outcome. Am J Surg Pathol. 2015;39(1):109–15. https://doi.org/10.1097/PAS.0000000000000320. PubMed PMID: 25229767; PubMed Central PMCID: PMC4267920.

Lebe B, Sarioğlu S, Sökmen S, Ellidokuz H, Füzün M, Küpelioğlu A. The clinical significance of p53, p21, and p27 expressions in rectal carcinoma. Appl Immunohistochem Mol Morphol. 2005;13(1):38–44. PubMed PMID: 15722792.

Müller MF, Ibrahim AE, Arends MJ. Molecular pathological classification of colorectal cancer. Virchows Arch. 2016;469(2):125–34. https://doi.org/10.1007/s00428-016-1956-3. Epub 2016 Jun 20. Review. PubMed PMID: 27325016; PubMed Central PMCID: PMC4978761.

Nagtegaal ID, Quirke P. Colorectal tumour deposits in the mesorectum and pericolon; a critical review. Histopathology. 2007;51(2):141–9. Epub 2007 May 26. Review. PubMed PMID: 17532768.

Nagtegaal ID, Tot T, Jayne DG, McShane P, Nihlberg A, Marshall HC, Påhlman L, Brown JM, Guillou PJ, Quirke P. Lymph nodes, tumor deposits, and TNM: are we getting better? J Clin Oncol. 2011;29(18):2487–92. https://doi.org/10.1200/JCO.2011.34.6429. Epub 2011 May 9. PubMed PMID: 21555695.

Puppa G, Ueno H, Kayahara M, Capelli P, Canzonieri V, Colombari R, Maisonneuve P, Pelosi G. Tumor deposits are encountered in advanced colorectal cancer and other adenocarcinomas: an expanded classification with implications for colorectal cancer staging system including a unifying concept of in-transit metastases. Mod Pathol. 2009;22(3):410–5. https://doi.org/10.1038/modpathol.2008.198. Epub 2009 Jan 9. PubMed PMID: 19136930.

Qiu HB, Chen G, Keshari RP, Luo HY, Fang W, Qiu MZ, Zhou ZW, Xu RH. The extramural metastasis might be categorized in lymph node staging for colorectal cancer. BMC Cancer. 2011;11(1):414. PubMed PMID: 21943144; PubMed Central PMCID: PMC3190391.

Ratto C, Ricci R, Valentini V, Castri F, Parello A, Gambacorta MA, Cellini N, Vecchio FM, Doglietto GB. Neoplastic mesorectal microfoci (MMF) following neoadjuvant chemoradiotherapy: clinical and prognostic implications. Ann Surg Oncol. 2007;14(2):853–61. PubMed PMID: 17103068.

Rock JB, Washington MK, Adsay NV, Greenson JK, Montgomery EA, Robert ME, Yantiss RK, Lehman AM, Frankel WL. Debating deposits: an interobserver variability study of lymph nodes and pericolonic tumor deposits in colonic adenocarcinoma. Arch Pathol Lab Med. 2014;138(5):636–42. https://doi.org/10.5858/arpa.2013-0166-OA. Epub 2013 Jul 31. PubMed PMID: 23902577; PubMed Central PMCID: PMC3935980.

Rogers AC, Winter DC, Heeney A, Gibbons D, Lugli A, Puppa G, Sheahan K. Systematic review and meta-analysis of the impact of tumour budding in colorectal cancer. Br J Cancer. 2016;115(7):831–40. https://doi.org/10.1038/bjc.2016.274. Epub 2016 Sep 6. PubMed PMID: 27599041; PubMed Central PMCID: PMC5046217.

Shimada Y, Takii Y. Clinical impact of mesorectal extranodal cancer tissue in rectal cancer: detailed pathological assessment using whole-mount sections. Dis Colon Rectum. 2010;53(5):771–8. https://doi.org/10.1007/DCR.0b013e3181cf7fd8. PubMed PMID: 20389211.

Siegel RL, Miller KD, Fedewa SA, Ahnen DJ, Meester RG, Barzi A, Jemal A. Colorectal cancer statistics, 2017. CA Cancer J Clin. 2017;67(3):177–93. https://doi.org/10.3322/caac.21395. PubMed PMID: 28248415.

Sis B, Sarioglu S, Sokmen S, Sakar M, Kupelioglu A, Fuzun M. Desmoplasia measured by computer assisted image analysis: an independent prognostic marker in colorectal carcinoma. J Clin Pathol. 2005;58(1):32–8. PubMed PMID: 15623479; PubMed Central PMCID: PMC1770537.

Sobin LH, Gospodarowicz M, Wittekind C, editors. International Union Against Cancer TNM classification of malignant tumours. 7th ed. Hoboken, NJ: Wiley-Blackwell; 2009.

Sobin LH, Wittekind C. TNM classification of malignant tumours. 6th ed. Hoboken, NJ: Wiley; 2002.

Sobin LH, Wittekind C. UICC TNM classification of malignant tumours. 5th ed. New York: Wiley; 1997.

Sokmen S, Sarioglu S, Füzün M, Terzi C, Küpelioglu A, Aslan B. Prognostic significance of angiogenesis in rectal cancer: a morphometric investigation. Anticancer Res. 2001a;21(6B):4341–8. PubMed PMID: 11908689.

Sokmen S, Lebe B, Sarioglu S, Füzün M, Terzi C, Küpelioglu A, Ellidokuz H. Prognostic value of CD44 expression in colorectal carcinomas. Anticancer Res. 2001b;21(6A):4121–6. PubMed PMID: 11911305.

Song YX, Gao P, Wang ZN, Liang JW, Sun Z, Wang MX, Dong YL, Wang XF, Xu HM. Can the tumor deposits be counted as metastatic lymph nodes in the UICC TNM staging system for colorectal cancer? PLoS One. 2012;7(3):e34087. https://doi.org/10.1371/journal.pone.0034087. Epub 2012 Mar 26. PubMed PMID: 22461900; PubMed Central PMCID: PMC3312887.

Tuna B, Sökmen S, Sarioğlu S, Füzün M, Küpelioğlu A, Ellidokuz H. PS2 and HSP70 expression in rectal adenocarcinomas: an immunohistochemical investigation of 45 cases. Appl Immunohistochem Mol Morphol. 2006;14(1):31–6. PubMed PMID: 16540727.

Ueno H, Murphy J, Jass JR, Mochizuki H, Talbot IC. Tumour 'budding' as an index to estimate the potential of aggressiveness in rectal cancer. Histopathology. 2002;40(2):127–32. PubMed PMID: 11952856.

Ueno H, Mochizuki H, Hashiguchi Y, Ishiguro M, Miyoshi M, Kajiwara Y, Sato T, Shimazaki H, Hase K. Extramural cancer deposits without nodal structure in colorectal cancer: optimal categorization for prognostic staging. Am J Clin Pathol. 2007;127(2):287–94. PubMed PMID: 17210518.

Ueno H, Mochizuki H, Shirouzu K, Kusumi T, Yamada K, Ikegami M, Kawachi H, Kameoka S, Ohkura Y, Masaki T, Kushima R, Takahashi K, Ajioka Y, Hase K, Ochiai A, Wada R, Iwaya K, Nakamura T, Sugihara K. Study group for tumor deposits without lymph node structure in colorectal cancer projected by the Japanese Society for cancer of the colon and rectum. Multicenter study for optimal categorization of extramural tumor deposits for colorectal cancer staging. Ann Surg. 2012;255(4):739–46. https://doi.org/10.1097/SLA.0b013e31824b4839. PubMed PMID: 22395093.

Yabata E, Udagawa M, Okamoto H. Effect of tumor deposits on overall survival in colorectal cancer patients with regional lymph node metastases. J Rural Med. 2014;9(1):20–6. https://doi.org/10.2185/jrm.2880. Epub 2014 Mar 7. PubMed PMID: 25648159; PubMed Central PMCID: PMC4310051.

Yamano T, Semba S, Noda M, Yoshimura M, Kobayashi M, Hamanaka M, Beppu N, Yano A, Tsukamoto K, Matsubara N, Tomita N. Prognostic significance of classified extramural tumor deposits and extracapsular lymph node invasion in T3-4 colorectal cancer: a retrospective single-center study. BMC Cancer. 2015;15:859. https://doi.org/10.1186/s12885-015-1885-6. PubMed PMID: 26545360; PubMed Central PMCID: PMC4635537.

Tumor Deposits in Gastric Cancer

4

Gastric carcinomas are frequent tumors with poor prognosis. They are the fifth most common cancer following lung, breast, colorectum, and prostate carcinomas and are twice more frequent in males. They are the third most frequent cause of cancer-related deaths. They have a geographic distribution, most frequent in the Far East, forming a triangle ending up at eastern Europe (http://globocan.iarc.fr/old/FactSheets/cancers/stomach-new.asp). The incidence of the disease decreased, and prognosis has improved during the last 40 years. One of the reasons for this change is the introduction of endoscopic equipment allowing early detection of tumors and dysplastic lesions as well as the recognition of the role of *Helicobacter pylori* in gastric carcinogenesis. However, gastric cancer is still a major health problem worldwide, and further prognostic and predictive factors are required for improving prognosis which is still poor. Many factors have been evaluated as prognostic markers in gastric carcinomas including tumor deposits or extranodal metastasis (EM). These lesions are focal aggregates of adenocarcinoma, discontinuous with the adenocarcinoma and showing no evidence of a lymph node morphology (Figs. 4.1, 4.2, and 4.3). The gastric carcinoma classifications, prognostic factors, and the importance of TDs will be briefly summarized.

Morphologic and Molecular Classifications of the Gastric Carcinomas and Prognostic Features

Histopathological classification of gastric carcinoma cases is difficult. Many architectural patterns and different types of cells may be seen, and it is not easy to apply the diagnostic criteria for tumor typing. The World Health Organization (WHO) classification includes a set of adenocarcinomas, but still Lauren's classification is used frequently by pathologists either alone or along with the WHO classification.

© Springer International Publishing AG 2018
S. Sarioglu, *Tumor Deposits*, https://doi.org/10.1007/978-3-319-68582-3_4

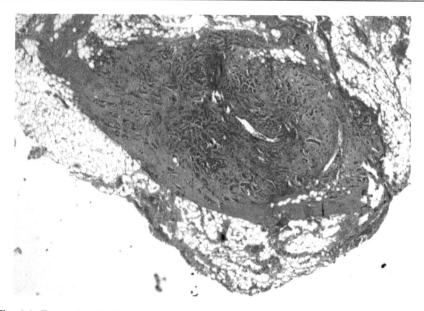

Fig. 4.1 Tumor deposit from a gastric carcinoma with partially irregular contours, probably related to a vessel (H&E, Original magnification, ×10)

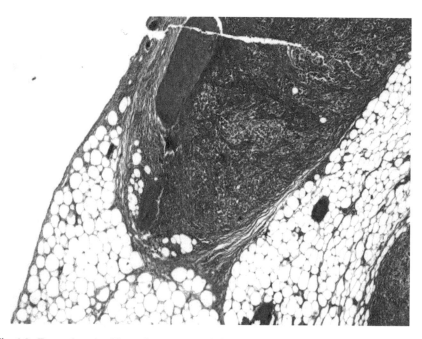

Fig. 4.2 Tumor deposit with regular contours; this figure may mimic a metastatic lymph node, but inside the tumor mass, there is a big peripheral nerve section not consistent with a lymph node structure (H&E, original magnification ×10)

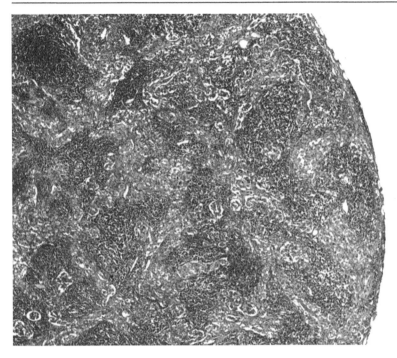

Fig. 4.3 Metastatic lymph node different from the lesions at Figs. 4.1 and 4.2. In this particular lesion, the metastatic tumor from a diffuse gastric carcinoma case is filling the sinusoids of the lymph node obscuring the normal morphology (H&E, original magnification ×20)

Lauren's classification (Lauren 1965), which was proposed in 1965, is simple but effective including only three types:

– Intestinal
– Diffuse
– Mixed

The latest WHO classification proposed different types of carcinomas (http://www.cap.org/ShowProperty?nodePath=/UCMCon/Contribution%20 Folders/WebContent/pdf/cp-stomach14-protocol.pdf):

– Papillary adenocarcinoma (Fig. 4.4)
– Tubular adenocarcinoma
– Mucinous adenocarcinoma
– Poorly cohesive carcinomas (include diffuse and signet-ring cell carcinoma) (Figs. 4.5 and 4.6)
– Mixed carcinoma

Rare variants:

– Adenosquamous carcinoma (Fig. 4.7)
– Carcinoma with lymphoid stroma
– Hepatoid adenocarcinoma (Figs. 4.8 and 4.9)

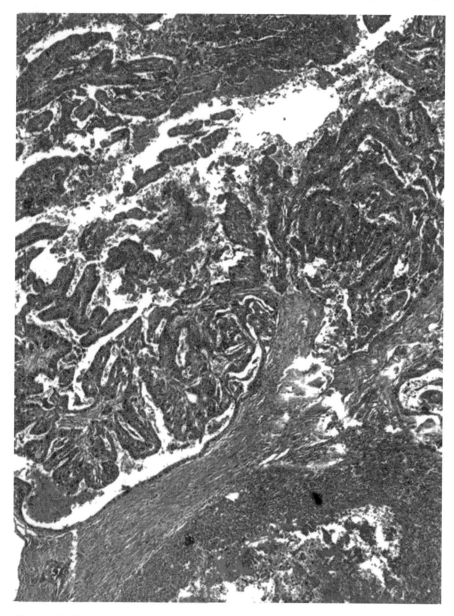

Fig. 4.4 Papillary gastric carcinoma (H&E, original magnification ×10)

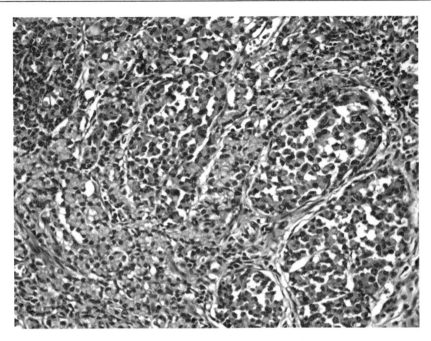

Fig. 4.5 Diffuse gastric carcinoma (H&E, original magnification ×20)

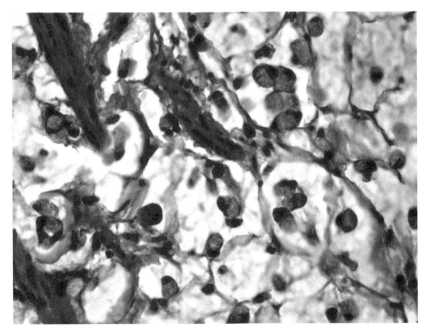

Fig. 4.6 Signet-ring carcinoma. Although the cells are floating in mucin, this case should not be classified as mucinous carcinoma if more than 50% of the tumor cells have the signet-ring cell morphology (H&E, original magnification ×40)

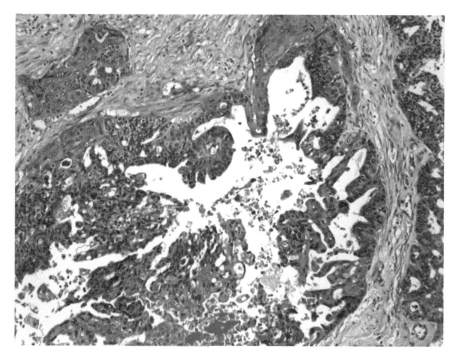

Fig. 4.7   Adenosquamous carcinoma (H&E, original magnification ×20)

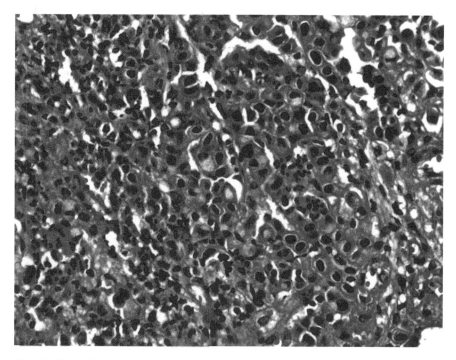

Fig. 4.8   Hepatoid adenocarcinoma, note relatively large cytoplasm (H&E, original magnification ×20)

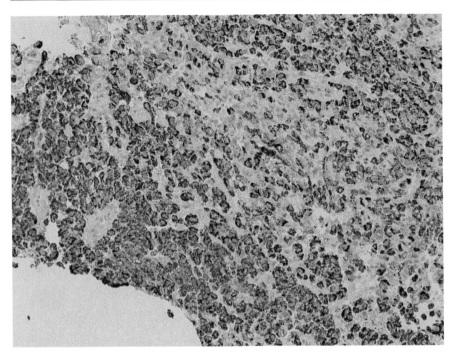

Fig. 4.9 Cytoplasmic hepatocyte-A expression, hepatoid gastric adenocarcinoma (immunohisto-chemistry, HEPA, original magnification ×100)

- Squamous cell carcinoma
- Undifferentiated carcinoma
- Neuroendocrine carcinoma (large-cell and small-cell neuroendocrine carcinoma, mixed adenoneuroendocrine carcinoma) (Fig. 4.10)

Goseki N et al.'s (1992) classification depends upon tubule formation and intracellular mucin content. Cases were divided into four groups, according to the findings in 200 autopsy cases with gastric carcinoma:

Group I: tubular differentiation, well; mucus in the cytoplasm, poor (associated with liver metastasis)
Group II: tubular differentiation, well; mucus in the cytoplasm, rich
Group III: tubular differentiation, poor; mucus in the cytoplasm, poor (associated with frequent bone marrow metastasis)
Group IV: tubular differentiation, poor; mucus in the cytoplasm, rich (associated with lymph node metastasis, direct invasion to the other organs, and peritonitis carcinomatosa)

According to the Cancer Genome Atlas Research Network (TCGA) proposal of molecular classification of gastric carcinomas, four groups were established (Cancer Genome Atlas Research Network 2014; Riquelme et al. 2015):

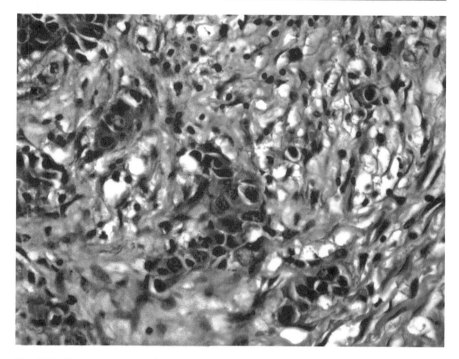

Fig. 4.10 Neuroendocrine carcinoma with signet-ring cells. For a definitive diagnosis of this rare case, positivity to neuroendocrine markers CD56, synaptophysin, or chromogranin-A is required (H&E, original magnification ×40)

EBV-Associated DNA Hypermethylation

Gastric carcinomas were associated with Epstein-Barr virus (EBV) in 9% of the cases (Figs. 4.11 and 4.12). Extreme CpG island methylator phenotype (CIMP) was identified as a distinct feature. All tumors had CDKN2A (p16) promoter hyper-methylation, but did not have MLH1 hypermethylation; the positivity of the latter one is a feature of microsatellite instability (MSI)-associated cancers. PIK3CA mutations were found in 80% of EBV-associated carcinomas and were identified at different sites of the gene in contrast to the non-EBV-associated carcinomas, whose mutations were most frequently located at exon 20 and mutated in 3–42% of the cases.

Microsatellite Instability

This group of cases was reported to be between 15 and 55% of the gastric carcinomas. At the TCGA series, 21% of these cases were of this type and more frequent in older females. The frequency may be related to the number of foci analyzed. This group of cases was associated with CIMP and MLH1 hypermethylation as well as

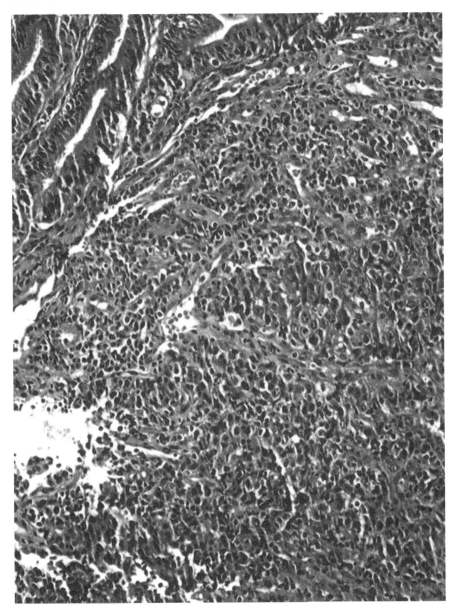

Fig. 4.11 Gastric carcinoma with diffuse pattern and distinct lymphocyte infiltration, typical morphology of EBV-associated tumors (H&E, original magnification ×20)

hypermutation. Elevated expression of mitotic network components was noted. Mutations were frequent including PIK3CA, ERBB3, ERBB2, and EGFR as well as other hotspot site mutations. MSI-high tumors were associated with intestinal-type adenocarcinomas and relatively better prognosis, while MSI-low tumors and

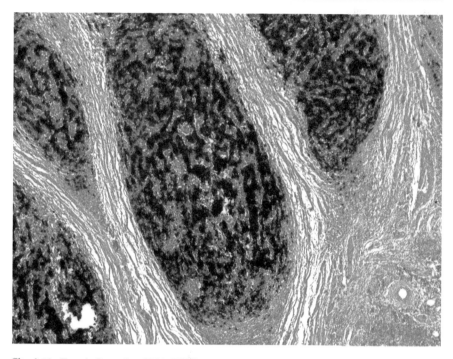

Fig. 4.12 Epstein-Barr virus RNA (EBER) chromogenic in situ hybridization (CISH) of the neoplasm in Fig. 4.11 (EBER CISH, original magnification ×20)

MSI-stable cases were associated with worse prognosis. MSI was thought to be related to the genes associated with cell cycle control.

Genomically Stable Tumors

The TCGA study identified this type in 20% of the cases and in younger patients. The diffuse type was predominant with rare p53 mutations and low degree of aneuploidy.

CDH1 germline mutations which are associated with hereditary gastric carcinoma were found to be associated with poor prognosis and diffuse phenotype. However, another group of cases, associated with comparatively better prognosis, was associated with RHOA pathway mutations and again altered cell adhesion.

Chromosomally Unstable Tumors

Nearly half of the cases was of this type and gastroesophageal junction was the frequent location. p53, ARID1A, k-RAS, RNF43, ERBB2, and APC gene mutations as well as aneuploidy were features of this type of tumors. EGFR amplification was frequent in this group. Frequent amplifications of genes encoding tyrosine kinase receptors, as well as cell cycle mediators, present opportunities in order to find targets of therapies.

There are targeted therapeutics against EGFR/ERBB2, VEGF, PI3K/AKT/mTOR, and HGF/MET pathways.

Prognostic Factors in Gastric Carcinomas

Gastric carcinomas may spread by three routes: by the lymphatics to the lymph nodes at the greater and lesser curvature and from there to the porta hepatis and para-aortic nodes or the left supraclavicular lymph node (Virchow's node), by the blood vessels to the liver and then lungs and other sites, or by the transperitoneal route resulting in peritoneal dissemination sometimes ending up at the ovaries giving rise to Krukenberg tumor and metastatic signet-ring cell carcinoma to the ovaries, in which case the most frequent site is the gastric carcinoma. However among these pathways, one additional route by tumor deposits has been described for gastric carcinomas, and this type of spread is also a poor prognostic factor.

The histopathological classifications and tumor grade do not provide prognostic information if the cases are stage matched. Tumor stage, lymph node stage, lymphovascular invasion and perineural invasion, and surgical margins are among the criteria that are required to be presented in pathology reports due their prognostic value (http://www.cap.org/ShowProperty?nodePath=/UCMCon/Contribution%20Folders/WebContent/pdf/cp-stomach14-protocol.pdf). Older age (over 70), proximal location, high levels of carcinoembryonic antigen (CEA), and CA19-9 are among the poor prognostic factors (Shiraishi et al. 2007). Early gastric carcinoma includes the cases which are only at the mucosa and submucosa, and even if these cases have lymph node metastasis, favorable prognosis might be expected, and the 5-year survival rates are over 90% (Hu et al. 2012).

The number of metastatic lymph nodes or pN stage is important in predicting prognosis like the pT stage. Tumor budding and single-cell invasion were found to be poor prognostic markers in gastric adenocarcinomas as well as micropapillary pattern (Fig. 4.13) which was suggested to be a feature at least partially related to tumor budding. In contrast to tumor budding, micropapillary pattern includes more than five cells and may be seen both at the invasive part and inside the tumor. MUC1 expression and decrease in E-cadherin expression are among the features of micropapillary morphology (Che K 2017, Zhang S 2016).

Considering the molecular classification of gastric carcinoma mentioned above, an important topic is HER2 gene amplification for both pathologists and oncologists. HER2 evaluation will be further detailed in this session.

HER2: A Predictive Biomarker in Gastric Carcinoma

HER2 is a proto-oncogene and a member of the epidermal growth factor family (EGFR). It is located on chromosome 17 that encodes a 185-kd tyrosine kinase receptor, whose phosphorylation initiates many types of signaling pathways, which lead to cell proliferation, differentiation, and apoptosis. The Human Genome Organization (HUGO) Nomenclature Committee (HGNC) approves the usage of ERBB2, CD340, HER2, and NEU as synonyms.

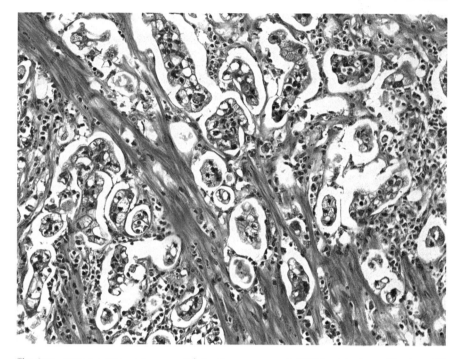

Fig. 4.13 Micropapillary pattern associated with poor prognosis (H&E, original magnification ×40)

HER2 gene is expressed in normal epithelial cells, and amplification and/or over-expression of this gene has been reported in up to one third of breast cancers as well as gastric cancers, but it may be overexpressed in many types of carcinomas (Kupelioglu et al. 1995a, b; Ozer et al. 2000). Among these some are squamous and some are non-squamous cell carcinomas.

The studies about the HER2 overexpression in gastric carcinomas and its relation with disease prognosis started a few decades ago. Overexpression of c-erbB2 was described as a poor prognostic marker associated with poor survival in gastric carcinomas (Yonemura et al. 1991, Jain et al. 1991). The histopathological type and gastric tumor location were identified among the factors influencing c-erbB2 expression (Albino et al. 1995). c-erbB2 expression and HER2 gene amplification were identified as independent poor prognostic factors in many series (Allgayer et al. 2000, García et al. 2003, Park et al. 2006).

Meanwhile the advances in breast carcinoma treatment were getting fruitful. Treatment with monoclonal antibody against HER2, Herceptin or trastuzumab, which inhibits signal transduction and induces cellular toxicity, was being applied, and better prognosis was achieved with the addition of this drug in HER2-positive breast carcinoma cases (Slamon et al. 2001, Piccart-Gebhart et al. 2005, Park et al. 2006). Although many types of tumors overexpress c-erbB2, the therapeutic efficacy of trastuzumab is only approved in gastric and/or gastroesophageal adenocarcinomas following breast carcinomas. However, the immunohistochemical scoring for gastric carcinomas is slightly different from the breast carcinoma cases which will be detailed in the "Immunohistochemistry" section (Hofmann et al. 2008).

Trastuzumab for Gastric Cancer (ToGA Trial) (Bang YJ 2010)

ToGA trial was an important cornerstone in gastric or gastroesophageal carcinoma treatment. The prognostic value of the combination treatment with trastuzumab with chemotherapy was evaluated in an open-label, randomized study; 122 centers from 24 countries participated. 3665 patients were included, and only 810 (22.10%) were positive for c-erbB2 overexpression by either immunohistochemistry or in situ hybridization (ISH). Having systemic diseases and/or previous chemotherapy was among the criteria for exclusion, and 594 patients were included in the trial and 584 completed the trial.

Chemotherapy protocol was as follows: Each of the six cycles was 3 weeks.

– Capecitabine 1000 mg/m^2 (oral twice a day for 14 days) 1-week rest
– Fluorouracil 800 mg/m^2 per day (continuous IV infusion; 1st–5th day of each cycle)
– Cisplatin 80 mg/m^2 on day 1 (IV infusion, 1st day of each cycle)

Trastuzumab protocol was as follows:

– IV infusion 8 mg/kg (1st day first cycle)
– IV infusion 6 mg/kg (1st day of the other cycles)

The overall survival was more than 2 months longer in patients who received trastuzumab and chemotherapy ($n = 298$) compared to the patients who received chemotherapy alone ($n = 290$). The adverse events were not significantly different for groups receiving trastuzumab, and following ToGA trial, trastuzumab in combination with chemotherapy is introduced as a new treatment option with prolonged survival for advanced gastric and gastroesophageal carcinoma.

Methods for Evaluation of HER2 Amplification

For a gastric carcinoma patient, having an option for targeted therapy for gastric cancer depends upon HER2 amplification. Trastuzumab does not prolong survival in patients who do not have HER2 overexpression. This resulted in the requirement for diagnostic molecular pathological evaluation for HER2 overexpression. Like many types of immunohistochemical and molecular pathological analysis tissue fixation, tissue processing and staining and/or hybridization procedures may affect the results, and procedures must be applied very carefully in order to avoid overtreatment or undertreatment. The tissue sections should not be thicker than 4 µm (Rüschoff J et al. 2010).

Immunohistochemistry

The HER2 expression interpretation method for gastric carcinomas is modified from breast carcinoma, after evaluation of the cases comparing ISH and immunohistochemistry results. There is more than one type of tissue for this testing HER2 overexpression, including biopsy specimens, gastrectomy, and/or esophagostomy specimens; furthermore metastatic tumor tissue may also be tested for this purpose. There are different criteria for these tissues.

The positive staining in breast carcinoma cases requires the positive membranous staining at the cell border including the luminal one. On the other hand, for gastric carcinomas, some of the cases with cell-positive staining at each border including basal and lateral but excluding luminal border were found to have HER2 amplification by ISH (Hofmann et al. 2008). With this finding, the HER2 positivity in gastric carcinomas has different criteria from the breast carcinomas, and luminal staining is not required. The positivity is semiquantitatively scored as negative, +, ++, and +++ (Figs. 4.14 and 4.15).

HER2 IHC biopsy interpretation (Bang YJ 2010): For reliable evaluation, the biopsy should be fixed at least for 6 hours in phosphate-buffered formalin solution, but the fixation should not be longer than 48 h. Underfixation, fixation for less than 6 h, may result in false-positive results. The period following biopsy till fixation should be as short as possible; the tissue should be fixed immediately.

−: If no staining is observed.

+: If faint positivity is observed at some of the cells. The positive cell percentage is not important. If the membranous staining can only be seen at ×40 magnification, the result should be +.

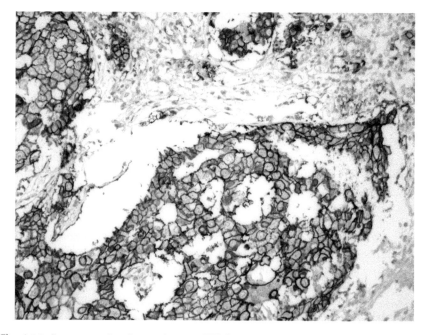

Fig. 4.14 Strong cytoplasmic membranous HER2 expression. HER2 expression is more frequently observed in carcinomas of the intestinal adenocarcinoma morphology (IHC, original magnification ×40)

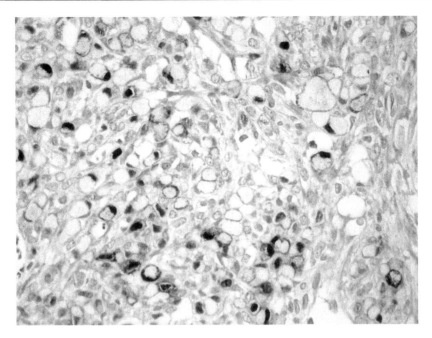

Fig. 4.15 Rarely the diffuse adenocarcinomas and signet-ring carcinomas may be positive for HER2 expression (IHC, original magnification ×40)

++: Mild to moderate membranous staining of cancer cell clusters. This category should be considered if the positive staining can be seen at ×10–×20 magnification.

+++: Strong membranous positivity of cancer cells making up five or more cells. If the positive staining can be seen at ×4 magnification, +++ result should be the diagnosis.

HER2 IHC radical surgical specimen interpretation (Bang YJ 2010): Only cytoplasmic, nuclear, only basal membranous, or only luminal staining should not be interpreted as positive.

Intratumoral heterogeneity of HER2 amplification is well known, and at the surgical specimen, larger tumor areas may be evaluated, possibly allowing observation of the amplification better. It is well known that gastric tumors with intestinal adenocarcinoma morphology have more HER2 overexpression compared with cases with weakly cohesive and/or signet-ring cell morphology. This is true for individual tumors having both intestinal and diffuse adenocarcinoma regions; again HER2 amplification is more frequently observed in tumor areas with the former morphology. Tissue block selected for IHC analysis should better have the most amount of tumor cells and areas with intestinal type of adenocarcinoma morphology.

In surgical specimens, the results should be interpreted as:

−: If less than 10% of cells are positive

+: If more than 10% of cells are positive with a faint membranous staining or partial membranous staining

++: If more than 10% of the tumor cells are weak to moderately positive in a complete, basolateral, or lateral membranous pattern of staining

+++: If more than 10% of the tumor cells are strongly positive in a complete, basolateral, or lateral membranous pattern of staining

The microscopic magnification applications described for biopsy specimens may be used also for the surgical specimens.

In Situ Hybridization

There are different options about the application of ISH for HER2 amplification. Both chromogenic or silver ISH and fluorescent ISH may be used. We prefer silver ISH (SISH). This method allows easier comparison of the IHC-stained tissue with the section where SISH is applied and cell counting at the tumor areas with the strongest HER2 IHC positivity.

One method is only testing the HER2 gene copy number with a single probe. The number reflects the amplification. The more frequently preferred method is dual ISH for chromosome 17 in which the HER2 gene is located, in a single section, using chromogens in different colors or silver. Counting the number of dots in different colors in 20 cells gives the following information:

– Number of chromosome 17
– HER2 gene copy numbers
– The ratio of these numbers (HER2 gene copy numbers/number of chromosome 17)

During the microscopic evaluation, there are many things to be careful about, including:

– Overlapping nuclei, nuclei with only one color staining, or nuclei without any staining should not be counted.
– Adjacent signals should be counted as one; for them to be counted as two, there should be a distance between them as big as the signals.
– In cases with high amplification of HER2 gene, the signals may make clusters; then the pathologist has to make an estimation about the possible number of signals making up the cluster. The diameter of single signals at the cell or neighbor stromal cells may help the estimation of the number.

If the ratio of HER2/Chr17 is less than or equal to 1.8, the result is accepted as negative for HER2 amplification, and if more than 2.2, then the result is positive for HER2 amplification. For cases with results in between, counting 20 more cells is recommended. In this case, if the ratio of HER2/Chr17 is less than 2, the result should be accepted as negative, and if equal to or more than 2, a positive result should be accepted (Fig. 4.16).

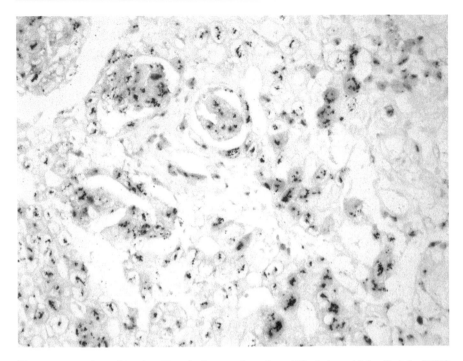

Fig. 4.16 HER2 amplification. Note the increased number of *black dots* which reflect the HER2 gene. Chromosome 17 is seen as red dots (dual in situ hybridization, original magnification ×40)

In some cases, Chr17 per cell may be less than 1, and deletion of HER2 gene should be considered. If very high numbers of Chr17 are observed like more than 6/ per cell, this may be due to amplification of the whole chromosome. In this case, even if the ratio of HER2/Chr17 is less than 2.2, still there will be HER2 amplification and the result should be positive.

HER2 ISH interpretation requires expertise, and pathologists should carry out this work always in conjunction with the hematoxylin and eosin slides and HER2 IHC-stained tissue sections.

The Diagnostic Combination of IHC and ISH for HER2 Amplification

It may seem logical to perform only ISH for the analysis of HER2 amplification. However, ISH is both more laborious and expensive than IHC, and there are other limitations. Even if there is amplification of a gene, there may not be the expression of the gene and no protein may be produced. In this case, targeting an amplified gene will not result in any prognostic advantage. It is recommended that IHC should be followed by ISH. In cases with negative or + HER2 IHC results, ISH is not recommended; the case is accepted as negative for HER2 amplification. If IHC HER2 expression is +++, again ISH is not recommended; the case is accepted as positive for HER2 amplification. It is only for cases with ++ IHC HER2 expression that HER2 ISH is recommended. Still there are many centers performing IHC and ISH for all cases or cases with ++/+++ HER2 IHC results.

The Incidence of HER2 Amplification in Gastric and Gastroesophageal Carcinoma Cases

HER2 protein overexpression identified by IHC may be reported as only +++ or ++/+++ in different series. In a review article, the percentage of ++/+++ cases ranged from 8.2 to 29.5. The positivity of HER2 amplification ranged from 9 to 27.1% by FISH and even as high as 36.6% by CISH (Boku 2014). In a series of 957 cases, Fan et al. (2013) reported +++ HER2 expression in 10.72% of the proximal and 0.81% of the distal cases, 17.6% of the low-grade and 0.26% of the high-grade cases, as well as 14.79% of the cases with intestinal morphology and 0.80% of the cases with diffuse histopathological morphology. For cases with distant metastatic disease, the HER2 IHC +++ results were as high as 36.36%, and for nonmetastatic cases, this was only 0.89% (Fan et al. 2013). Laboissiere et al. reported +++, ++, +, and negative results in 10.5, 8.1, 0.56, and 81.4% of the cases in a series of 124 cases, respectively, and only detected HER2 positivity by ISH in +++ HER2 IHC-positive cases. They observed HER2 overexpression and amplification in 10% of the distal and 12.5% of the proximal gastric and esophagogastric junctional cases. The cases with intestinal morphology showed HER2 overexpression in 18% of the cases, and none of the diffuse gastric carcinoma cases were positive (Laboissiere et al. 2015).

The gastric biopsy and surgery specimens were compared for HER2 positivity in a series of 61 cases by Pirrelli et al. (2013) The same results were achieved in both types of specimens in 91% of the cases. The false-negative three cases showed intra-tumoral heterogeneity, and the false-positive cases showed staining of HER2 IHC without HER2 gene amplification.

These results may be summarized as follows: *HER2* overexpression and *HER2* gene amplification, poor prognostic markers for gastric adenocarcinomas, are more frequent in proximal gastric cases and in cases with low-grade differentiation and intestinal adenocarcinoma morphology as well as distant metastatic disease (Erdamar S et al. 2014, Pirrelli M et al. 2013, Fan et al. 2013, Boku 2014, Laboissiere et al. 2015). If possible, surgical specimens should be preferred for evaluation of HER2 overexpression and amplification.

Implications for Treatment

According to the recent guidelines, HER2-positive, advanced, or metastatic gastric adenocarcinoma patients should be treated with trastuzumab in combination with chemotherapy. A combination of cisplatin and fluoropyrimidine may be selected, but anthracyclines are not recommended to be used with trastuzumab (Ajani et al. 2013).

There are still some questions to be answered about the use of trastuzumab in gastric carcinoma patients: Is trastuzumab an option for patients who progress under chemotherapy? What should be done for patients who progress under trastuzumab and chemotherapy? Should we only change chemotherapy and keep on with trastuzumab? Would addition of trastuzumab adjuvant therapy for HER2-overexpressing resectable gastric cancer be beneficial? All of these questions are under investigation in different trials. Other anti-HER2-targeted therapies are also under investigation, and dual HER2 inhibition therapies may become better treatment options soon (Ajani et al. 2013, Gomez-Martín C 2014).

Proposed Mechanisms and Morphology of Tumor Deposits in Gastric Carcinomas

Much attention was focused on the mechanism of TD formation in colorectal carcinomas; however, the information about the gastric carcinoma cases is sparse. The researchers mostly focused on the importance of TDs as prognostic factors and their roles in TNM classifications. Some possible proposed mechanisms for TD formation in gastric carcinoma patients were as follows:

Lymphatic and venous communication was described as a result of the obstruction of the lymph nodes by the neoplastic metastatic cells. Jiang et al. (2014) suggested that the TDs were associated with extranodal spread from the metastatic lymph nodes and resulted in peritoneal dissemination and distant metastasis.

In the series of Etoh et al. (2006), considering the increased incidence of peritonitis carcinomatosa in gastric carcinoma cases with TDs, the authors suggested that direct spread of tumor cells from high-grade tumors and/or extranodal deposits occurred subsequent to lymph node metastasis. Furthermore lymphaticovenous communication and obstructed lymphatics were discussed in the mechanism.

In the series of Lee et al. (2013), TDs were grouped into five morphological types, and the separate nodular pattern was suggested to be the end stage of carcinoma obscuring the origin. Perivascular pattern was explained as the vessel invasion by carcinoma outside the adventitia. The other patterns were explained as lymphatic, perineural, and endovascular invasion.

Classifications of Tumor Deposits in Gastric Carcinomas

The classification of TDs in gastric carcinomas has been a dilemma for many years, like in colorectal carcinomas. Including these lesions under T, N, and M categories has been proposed. The American Joint Committee on Cancer (AJCC)/International Union Against Cancer (UICC) classification, 5th and 6th edition, regarded these lesions as metastatic lymph nodes if the lesions had smooth contours, and if the lesions did not have smooth contours, then the lesions should be included under primary tumors, that is to say pT stage. At the 7th edition, metastatic nodules in the fat tissue adjacent to a gastric carcinoma should be accepted as lymph node metastasis, but the deposits implanted on the peritoneal surfaces should be considered as distant metastasis, and there were no further changes at the last classification (2017) (Sobin and Wittekind 1997, 2002; Sobin et al. 2010, Brierley J et al. 2017).

Etoh et al. (2006) evaluated the tumor deposits or extranodal deposits in 1023 gastric carcinoma cases and described tumor deposits simply as follows:

> "Presence of cancer cells in soft tissue that was discontinuous with the primary lesion or in perinodal soft tissue distinct from the lymph node."

Wang et al. (2011) did not specify the criteria they used for referring a tumor mass as TD and did not classify TDs into subcategories.

In the series of Sun et al. (2012), TDs were evaluated according to the TNM7 criteria for colorectal carcinoma cases.

In a series of 635 gastric carcinoma cases, Lee et al. (2013) evaluated the cases according to these criteria, stating that *"TD were defined as macroscopic or microscopic depositions of carcinoma in perigastric fat tissue without any residual lymph node structures,"* and classified these lesions into five groups regarding the origin and the morphology as follows:

- Separate nodular pattern
- Perivascular pattern
- Perineural pattern
- Lymphatic pattern
- Endovascular pattern

In our series of gastric carcinomas, TDs were classified as perivascular, perineural, lymphatic, and mixed patterns, and the diameters of the TDs were measured (Ersen et al. 2014).

In the study by Jiang et al. (2014), the tumor deposits were defined as cancer cells in soft tissue that was discontinuous with the primary tumor or in peri-stomach soft tissue distinct from a lymph node.

Prognostic Studies on Tumor Deposits in Gastric Carcinomas

In a series of 1023 gastric carcinoma cases, Etoh et al. (2006) reported that the tumor deposits were identified in 146 (14.3%) of the cases. TDs were associated with poor prognostic histopathological factors as well as poor survival. TDs were more frequent in large-diameter, infiltrative, and high-pT-stage tumors. Peritoneal and, liver metastasis as well as vascular and lymphatic invasion were more frequent in cases with TDs. Overall survival was poor for the cases with TDs, and the hazard ratio for these cases was 1.82. Only pT and metastatic lymph node positivity and TDs were independent prognostic factors. Peritoneal carcinomatosis was positive in 2.3% of the cases without tumor deposits, but it was positive in 40.4% of the cases with TDs. According to these findings, Etoh et al. suggested that TDs should be included in the classification of gastric carcinomas.

Wang et al. (2011) found TDs in 13.3% of the patients in a series of 1343 gastric carcinoma cases. They found TDs as poor and independent prognostic factors and named them as extramural metastasis (EM). The number of EMs was important in predicting prognosis. Five-year survival rates of patients who had 1, 2, and more than 3 EMs were 35.2%, 27.6%, and 6.8%, respectively, and the authors grouped the cases with 1–2 TDs as EM 1 and cases with TDs $\geq$ 3 as EM2. EM1 cases had a prognosis similar to N3 cases and EM2 cases had prognosis similar to T4 cases, and the authors suggested the incorporation of TDs to the TNM classification according to these findings.

Sun et al. (2012) evaluated 2998 patients and found TDs in 17.8% of the cases. In this series, a number of TDs were also evaluated. They identified TDs as poor prognostic markers, and they experimented stage migrations for N and T categories and found that they were more significant for T category and suggested that they should be classified as a form of serosal invasion and patients with TDs should receive adjuvant chemotherapy.

Lee et al. (2013) also identified TDs as poor prognostic markers. Of the 653 gastric carcinoma patients, 156 (23.9%) had TDs. TDs were found to be independent prognostic factors for overall survival (hazard ratio 2.089) and distant metastasis (hazard ratio: 4.803) in multivariate analysis. Morphologically different TD types were not different for survival parameters. Only 13 cases had TDs but no lymph node metastasis, and these cases had worse prognosis than the ones without TDs and lymph node metastasis. In contrast to the conclusions drawn by Sun et al. (2012) who suggested that the TDs should be changing the T stage, Lee HS et al. suggested that TDs should be calculated as metastatic lymph nodes and pN stage should be given according to the sum of metastatic lymph nodes and TDs.

In our series (Ersen et al. 2014) including 96 gastric carcinoma cases, TDs were identified in 23%. TDs were more frequent in intestinal type of carcinoma cases. TDs, the number of perilymphatic TDs and the diameter of perivascular TDs, pT and pN stage, vascular invasion, and positive surgical margins were features predicting recurrences. The number of lymph nodes and perilymphatic TDs, pT and pN stage, and perineural, vascular, and lymphatic invasion were important for overall survival.

In the series by Jiang et al. (2014), 642 (26.79%) of the gastric carcinoma cases had tumor deposits. TDs were significantly more frequent in cases with the primary tumor of more than 5 cm diameter, increased pT, lymph node metastasis, and peritoneal and distant recurrences. Depth of invasion, lymph node metastasis, and TDs were independent prognostic factors for overall survival, while lymph node metastasis, TDs, lymph node metastasis, and tumor size were independent prognostic factors for disease-free survival. Five-year overall free and disease-free survival rates were 48.1% and 17.4% and 44.5% and 14.3% for TD-negative and TD-positive cases, respectively. Also in this series, they incorporated pN stage and TDs making up a new classification named as pNE; the groups were as follows:

pNE0: pN0 and TD:0
pNE1: pN1 and TD:0
pNE2: pN2 and TD:0 of pN0 and TD:1 or TD $\geq$ 2

pNE3: pN1 and TD:1 or TD $\geq$ 2 or pN2 and TD:1 or TD $\geq$ 2
pNE4: pN3 and TD:0 and TD:1
pNE5: pN3 and TD $\geq$ 2

pN groups and pNE cases were both independent prognostic factors. The hazard ratio for pNE5 was 15.398. The 5-year survival rates for pNE1 to pNE5 were 77.7, 58.6, 40.0, 31.5, 14.7, and 2.8%, respectively.

Furthermore the peritoneal metastasis was significantly more frequent in cases with TDs with a hazard ratio of 2.448. Peritoneal recurrences were identified in 17 and 37.8% of the TD-negative and TD-positive cases, and TDs were the strongest factor for predicting peritoneal recurrence. Jiang N et al. suggested that intra-arterial, intravenous, and intraperitoneal chemotherapy should be considered in cases with TDs.

In the series of Yildiz et al. (2016), TDs were identified in 26.2% of the gastric carcinoma cases. In multivariate analysis, TDs were identified as independent prognostic markers, and TD-positive cases had 1.75-fold likelihood of developing recurrences, and the risk of death increased 1.99-fold.

In a series of 1457 gastric carcinomas, TDs were found in 133 (9.1%) of the cases (Chen et al. 2016). The TD-positive group had worse prognosis and more advanced carcinoma. For the cases in stages I, II, and III, TDs were independent prognostic factors. Cases with more than 2 TDs had larger tumor size and more advanced N stage than cases with 1 or 2 TDs. The number of TDs was an independent prognostic factor. The authors suggested that cases with more than 2 TDs should be grouped among TNM IV stage.

Discussion About TDs in Gastric Carcinomas

Gastric carcinomas are among the most important health problems. Identifying prognostic markers is very important for gastric carcinoma patients, as well as for patients of many other types of carcinomas.

Most of the studies about the TDs were carried out in colorectal carcinomas. Gastric carcinomas were also evaluated for TDs; the largest series about TDs following the colorectal carcinoma cases are the gastric carcinoma cases. Although much attention was focused on the types of TDs in colorectal carcinomas, these attempts are sparse in gastric carcinomas. Lee et al. (2013) and Ersen et al. (2014) classified the cases with TDs into morphological groups like perivascular and perineural patterns. There are no studies about the interobserver reliability in TDs in gastric carcinoma cases. The cases with TDs ranged from 9.1 to 26.79% in different series. This difference between the percentage of the TD-positive cases may be related to the applied criteria.

The results of all series are in favor of poor prognosis in gastric carcinomas with TDs (Etoh et al. 2006; Wang et al. 2011; Sun et al. 2012; Lee et al. 2013; Ersen et al. 2014; Jiang et al. 2014; Chen et al. 2016). The TDs are included among the metastatic lymph nodes in TNM staging manuals (http://globocan.iarc.fr/old/FactSheets/

cancers/stomach-new.asp; https://www.iarc.fr/en/publications/pdfs-online/pat-gen/bb2/bb2-chap3.pdf; http://www.cap.org/ShowProperty?nodePath=/UCMCon/Contribution%20Folders/WebContent/pdf/cp-stomach14-protocol.pdf). However, in different series, either the positivity of TDs or cases with two or more TDs were found to have worse prognosis compatible with stage IV cases, and it was proposed that they should be classified as such (Chen et al. 2016). Increased number of TDs is associated with poor prognosis, and grouping the cases into prognostic subtypes according to the number of TDs along with metastatic lymph nodes was proposed (Jiang et al. 2014), as well as the classification of cases with more than 2 TDs as stage IV disease (Chen et al. 2016).

Cases with TDs were found to be more frequently associated with peritoneal metastasis. In the series of Etoh et al. (2006), peritoneal metastasis was 20 times more frequent in cases with TDs. In the series by Jiang N et al., peritoneal metastasis was significantly more frequent in cases with TDs with a hazard ratio of 2.448. In this series, peritoneal metastasis was more than twice as common in cases with TDs, and TDs were found as the strongest predictive factor for peritoneal metastasis.

Series with considerable number of cases have been evaluated for the value of TDs in gastric carcinomas, but there is still no consensus about the final classification of these lesions in gastric carcinoma cases. Although, according to the last TNM classification, they are included among the pN category and counted as metastatic lymph nodes, reporting them in pathology reports as TDs should not be neglected. Considering the poor prognostic outcome and tendency for peritoneal metastasis, for the cases with TDs, the strongest treatment modalities should be selected.

References

Ajani JA, Bentrem DJ, Besh S, D'Amico TA, Das P, Denlinger C, Fakih MG, Fuchs CS, Gerdes H, Glasgow RE, Hayman JA, Hofstetter WL, Ilson DH, Keswani RN, Kleinberg LR, Korn WM, Lockhart AC, Meredith K, Mulcahy MF, Orringer MB, Posey JA, Sasson AR, Scott WJ, Strong VE, Varghese TK Jr, Warren G, Washington MK, Willett C, Wright CD, McMillian NR, Sundar H, National Comprehensive Cancer Network. Gastric cancer, version 2.2013: featured updates to the NCCN guidelines. J Natl Compr Cancer Netw. 2013;11(5):531–46.

Albino AP, Jaehne J, Altorki N, Blundell M, Urmacher C, Lauwers G, Niedzwiecki D, Kelsen DP. Amplification of HER-2/neu gene in human gastric adenocarcinomas: correlation with primary site. Eur J Surg Oncol. 1995;21(1):56–60.

Allgayer H, Babic R, Gruetzner KU, Tarabichi A, Schildberg FW, Heiss MM. c-erbB-2 is of independent prognostic relevance in gastric cancer and is associated with the expression of tumor-associated protease systems. J Clin Oncol. 2000;18(11):2201–9.

Bang Y-J, Van Cutsem E, Feyereislova A, Chung HC, Shen L, Sawaki A, Lordick F, Ohtsu A, Omuro Y, Satoh T, Aprile G, Kulikov E, Hill J, Lehle M, Rüschoff J, Kang Y-K. Trastuzumab in combination with chemotherapy versus chemotherapy alone for treatment of HER2-positive advanced gastric or gastro-oesophageal junction cancer (ToGA): a phase 3, open-label, randomised controlled trial. Lancet. 2010;376(9742):687–97.

Boku N. HER2-positive gastric cancer. Gastric Cancer. 2014;17(1):1–12.

Brierley J, Gospodarowicz M, Wittekind C. UICC TNM classification of malignant tumours. 8th ed. Chichester: Wiley; 2017.

Cancer Genome Atlas Research Network. Comprehensive molecular characterization of gastric adenocarcinoma. Nature. 2014;513(7517):202–9. https://doi.org/10.1038/nature13480. Epub 2014 Jul 23. PubMed PMID: 25079317; PubMed Central PMCID: PMC4170219.

Che K, Zhao Y, Qu X, Pang Z, Ni Y, Zhang T, Du J, Shen H. Prognostic significance of tumor budding and single cell invasion in gastric adenocarcinoma. Onco Targets Ther. 2017;10:1039–47. https://doi.org/10.2147/OTT.S127762. eCollection 2017. PubMed PMID: 28255247; PubMed Central PMCID: PMC5325090.

Chen XL, Zhao LY, Xue L, Xu YH, Zhang WH, Liu K, Chen XZ, Yang K, Zhang B, Chen ZX, Chen JP, Zhou ZG, Hu JK. Prognostic significance and the role in TNM stage of extranodal metastasis within regional lymph nodes station in gastric carcinoma. Oncotarget. 2016;7(41):67047–60. 10.18632/oncotarget.11478. PubMed PMID: 27563811; PubMed Central PMCID: PMC5341856.

Erdamar S, Kepil N, Dursun A, Ekinci O, Sagol S, Sarioglu S, Doganavsargil B, Sezak B, Ozdener F, Ustundag K. Epidemiologic study on HER2 (+) early/advanced stage gastric cancer: an evaluation on HER2 positivity in gastric and gastroesophageal junction cancers. Virchow Archiv. 2014;465(Suppl 1):S148.

Ersen A, Unlu MS, Akman T, Sagol O, Oztop I, Atila K, Bora S, Ellidokuz H, Sarioglu S. Tumor deposits in gastric carcinomas. Pathol Res Pract. 2014;210(9):565–70. https://doi.org/10.1016/j.prp.2014.03.006. Epub 2014 Mar 27. PubMed PMID: 24726262.

Etoh T, Sasako M, Ishikawa K, Katai H, Sano T, Shimoda T. Extranodal metastasis is an indicator of poor prognosis in patients with gastric carcinoma. Br J Surg. 2006;93(3):369–73. PubMed PMID: 16392106.

Fan XS, Chen JY, Li CF, Zhang YF, Meng FQ, Wu HY, Feng AN, Huang Q. Differences in HER2 over-expression between proximal and distal gastric cancers in the Chinese population. World J Gastroenterol. 2013;19(21):3316–23.

García I, Vizoso F, Martín A, Sanz L, Abdel-Lah O, Raigoso P, García-Muñiz JL. Clinical significance of the epidermal growth factor receptor and HER2 receptor in resectable gastric cancer. Ann Surg Oncol. 2003;10(3):234–41.

Gomez-Martín C, Lopez-Rios F, Aparicio J, Barriuso J, García-Carbonero R, Pazo R, Rivera F, Salgado M, Salud A, Vázquez-Sequeiros E, Lordick F. A critical review of HER2-positive gastric cancer evaluation and treatment: from trastuzumab, and beyond. Cancer Lett. 2014;351(1):30–40.

Goseki N, Takizawa T, Koike M. Differences in the mode of the extension of gastric cancer classified by histological type: new histological classification of gastric carcinoma. Gut. 1992;33(5):606–12. PubMed PMID: 1377153; PubMed Central PMCID: PMC1379287.

Hofmann M, Stoss O, Shi D, Büttner R, van de Vijver M, Kim W, Ochiai A, Rüschoff J, Henkel T. Assessment of a HER2 scoring system for gastric cancer: results from a validation study. Histopathology. 2008;52(7):797–805.

http://www.cap.org/ShowProperty?nodePath=/UCMCon/Contribution%20Folders/WebContent/pdf/cp-stomach14-protocol.pdf. Last accessed 18 May 2017.

Hu B, El Hajj N, Sittler S, Lammert N, Barnes R, Meloni-Ehrig A. Gastric cancer: classification, histology and application of molecular pathology. J Gastrointest Oncol. 2012;3(3):251–61. https://doi.org/10.3978/j.issn.2078-6891.2012.021. PubMed PMID: 22943016; PubMed Central PMCID: PMC3418539.

Jain S, Filipe MI, Gullick WJ, Linehan J, Morris RW. c-erbB-2 proto-oncogene expression and its relationship to survival in gastric carcinoma: an immunohistochemical study on archival material, hit. J Cancer. 1991;48:668–71.

Jiang N, Deng JY, Ding XW, Ke B, Liu N, Liang H. Node-extranodal soft tissue stage based on extranodal metastasis is associated with poor prognosis of patients with gastric cancer. J Surg Res. 2014;192(1):90–7. https://doi.org/10.1016/j.jss.2014.05.053. Epub 2014 May 23. PubMed PMID: 24953988.

Kupelioglu A, Sarioglu S, Atac G, Simsek I, Akpınar H, Ozen E. Immunohistochemical analysis of p53, cerbB2, PCNA expressions in gastric adenocarcinoma. Turkish J Neoplasia. 1995a;4(1):7–10.

Kupelioglu A, Sarioglu S, Atac G, Akpinar H, Ozen E. Immunohistochemical analysis of p53, cerbB2, PCNA expressions in colorectal adenocarcinoma. Turkish J Neoplasia. 1995b;4(11):11–5.

Laboissiere RS, Buzelin MA, Balabram D, De Brot M, Nunes CB, Rocha RM, Cabral MM, Gobbi H. Association between HER2 status in gastric cancer and clinicopathological features: a retrospective study using whole-tissue sections. BMC Gastroenterol. 2015;15:157.

Lauren P. The two histological main types of gastric carcinoma: diffuse and so-called intestinal-type carcinoma. An attempt at a histo-clinical classification. Acta Pathol Microbiol Scand. 1965;64:31–49. PubMed PMID: 14320675.

Lee HS, Lee HE, Yang HK, Kim WH. Perigastric tumor deposits in primary gastric cancer: implications for patient prognosis and staging. Ann Surg Oncol. 2013;20(5):1604–13. https://doi.org/10.1245/s10434-012-2692-9. Epub 2012 Nov 25. PubMed PMID: 23184289.

Ozer E, Sis B, Ozen E, Sakızlı M, Canda T, Sarioglu S. BRCA1, C-erbB-2, and H-ras gene expressions in young women with breast cancer—an immunohistochemical study. Appl Immunohistochem Mol Morphol. 2000;8(1):12–8.

Park DI, Yun JW, Park JH, Oh SJ, Kim HJ, Cho YK, Sohn CI, Jeon WK, Kim BI, Yoo CH, Son BH, Cho EY, Chae SW, Kim EJ, Sohn JH, Ryu SH, Sepulveda AR. HER-2/neu amplification is an independent prognostic factor in gastric cancer. Dig Dis Sci. 2006;51(8):1371–9.

Piccart-Gebhart MJ, Procter M, Leyland-Jones B, et al. Trastuzumab after adjuvant chemotherapy in HER2-positive breast cancer. N Engl J Med. 2005;353:1659–72.

Pirrelli M, Caruso ML, Di Maggio M, Armentano R, Valentini AM. Are biopsy specimens predictive of HER2 status in gastric cancer patients? Dig Dis Sci. 2013;58(2):397–404. doi:10.1007/s10620-012-2357-3. Epub 2012 Aug 24. PubMed PMID: 22918687.

Riquelme I, Saavedra K, Espinoza JA, Weber H, García P, Nervi B, Garrido M, Corvalán AH, Roa JC, Bizama C. Molecular classification of gastric cancer: towards a pathway-driven targeted therapy. Oncotarget. 2015;6(28):24750–79. 10.18632/oncotarget.4990. Review. PubMed PMID: 26267324; PubMed Central PMCID: PMC4694793.

Rüschoff J, Dietel M, Baretton G, Arbogast S, Walch A, Monges G, Chenard MP, Penault-Llorca F, Nagelmeier I, Schlake W, Höfler H, Kreipe HH. HER2 diagnostics in gastric cancer-guideline validation and development of standardized immunohistochemical testing. Virchows Arch. 2010;457(3):299–307.

Shiraishi N, Sato K, Yasuda K, Inomata M, Kitano S. Multivariate prognostic study on large gastric cancer. J Surg Oncol. 2007;96(1):14–8. Review. PubMed PMID: 17582596.

Slamon DJ, Leyland-Jones B, Shak S, et al. Use of chemotherapy plus a monoclonal antibody against HER2 for metastatic breast cancer that overexpresses HER2. N Engl J Med. 2001;344:783–92.

Sobin LH, Wittekind C. UICC TNM classification of malignant tumours. 5th ed. New York: Wiley; 1997.

Sobin LH, Wittekind C. TNM classification of malignant tumours. 6th ed. Hoboken, NJ: Wiley; 2002.

Sobin LH, Gospodarowicz MK, Wittekind C. TNM classification of malignant tumours. 7th ed. Hoboken, NJ: Wiley-Blackwell; 2010.

Sun Z, Wang ZN, Xu YY, Zhu GL, Huang BJ, Xu Y, Liu FN, Zhu Z, Xu HM. Prognostic significance of tumor deposits in gastric cancer patients who underwent radical surgery. Surgery. 2012;151(6):871–81. https://doi.org/10.1016/j.surg.2011.12.027. Epub 2012 Mar 3. PubMed PMID: 22386276.

Wang W, Li Y, Zhang Y, Yuan X, Xu D, Guan Y, Feng X, Chen Y, Sun X, Li W, Zhan Y, Zhou Z. Incorporation of extranodal metastasis of gastric carcinoma into the 7th edition UICC TNM staging system. PLoS One. 2011;6(6):e19557. https://doi.org/10.1371/journal.pone.0019557. Epub 2011 Jun 13. PubMed PMID: 21695186; PubMed Central PMCID: PMC3113802.

Yildiz B, Etiz D, Dal P, Junushova B, Pasaoglu O, Yilmaz E, Erkasap S, Dincer M. Tumor deposits: prognostic significance in gastric cancer patients. J BUON. 2016;21(6):1476–81. PubMed PMID: 28039711.

Yonemura Y, Ninomiya I, Yamaguchi A, Fushida S, Kimura H, Ohoyama S, et al. Evaluation of immunoreactivity for erbB-2 protein as a marker of poor short term prognosis in gastric cancer. Cancer Res. 1991;51:1034–8.

Zhang S, Zhang D, Yang Z, Zhang X. Tumor budding, micropapillary pattern, and polyploidy Giant cancer cells in colorectal cancer: current status and future prospects. Stem Cells Int. 2016;2016:4810734. Epub 2016 Oct 23. Review. PubMed PMID: 27843459; PubMed Central PMCID: PMC5097820.

Tumor Deposits in Esophageal Carcinomas

5

Esophageal carcinomas are relatively rare; nearly 1% of the newly diagnosed cases in the USA are of this type (1). Most frequent types of esophageal carcinomas are squamous cell carcinomas and adenocarcinomas. Esophageal squamous cell carcinomas (ESCC) were the most frequent type all around the world for many decades; however, since 1970, there is a decrease in ESCC, and the number of esophageal adenocarcinomas (EAC) is increasing in the Western world. These changes may be related to decreased tobacco and alcohol consumption leading to less frequent ESCC cases and obesity and gastroesophageal reflux disease (GERD) leading to the development of EAC.

Morphologic and Molecular Classifications of the Esophageal Carcinomas

ESCC cases are most frequently located at the middle esophagus, and they seem to develop due to diets low in vitamins and increased alcohol and tobacco consumption. Human papilloma virus infection is not proved as a factor for ESCC development (Jain and Dhingra 2017). Achalasia, an esophageal neurodegenerative motility disorder, is also associated with increased risk of ESCC, probably due to food stasis at the esophagus and chronic inflammation (O'Neill et al. 2013). Tylosis is a disease with high frequency of ESCC, and RHBDF2 (*tylosis esophageal cancer gene*) mutation is the underlying mechanism for this disease (Ellis et al. 2015). While classical ESCC are the most frequent type, SCC variants like basaloid SCC and verrucous carcinoma as well as carcinosarcoma (Cavallin et al. 2014) may be seen, which also have prognostic implications (Fig. 5.1).

The development of EAC is related to Barrett's esophagus, which is diagnosed by endoscopic and histopathological examination, characterized by columnar epithelium at the distal esophagus (Fig. 5.2). The most frequent type of EAC is the classical type, but mucinous and signet-ring types may also be seen (Fig. 5.3). If the epicenter of an adenocarcinoma is located within 5 cm to the esophageal or gastric

© Springer International Publishing AG 2018
S. Sarioglu, *Tumor Deposits*, https://doi.org/10.1007/978-3-319-68582-3_5

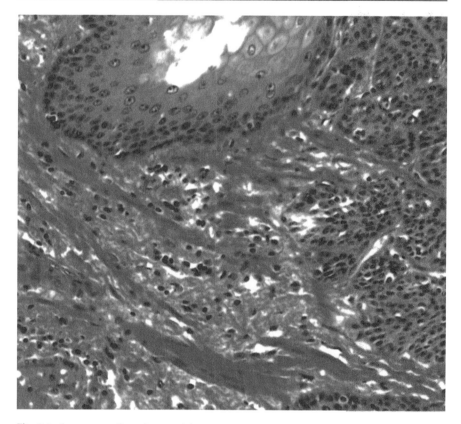

Fig. 5.1 Squamous cell carcinoma of the esophagus invasive to the muscular layer with keratinization (H&E, original magnification ×40)

side of the gastroesophageal junction, the tumor is named as gastroesophageal junction adenocarcinoma (Jain and Dhingra 2017).

The molecular analysis of esophageal SCC and adenocarcinoma cases was unveiled recently by the Cancer Genome Atlas Research Network Analysis Working Group (2017). The results revealed three molecular subclasses for ESCC cases:

ESCC1: This group was characterized by alterations in the NRF2 pathway, a regulator of adaptation to oxidative stressors like carcinogens and chemotherapy agents. This group had alteration in genes degrading NRF2 genes like NFE2L2. SOX2 and NRF2 amplifications were frequent. These features were like the SCC of the head and neck (Cancer Genome Atlas Research Network Analysis Working Group 2015). YAP1 amplification and VGLL4/ATG7 deletion were frequent, and these findings suggest the activation of Hippo.

ESCC2: NOTCH1 or ZNF750 mutations, PTEN or PIK3R1, KDM6A and KDM2D inactivations, CDK6 amplifications, and leukocyte infiltration were frequent in this group as well as increased levels of caspase 7 protein.

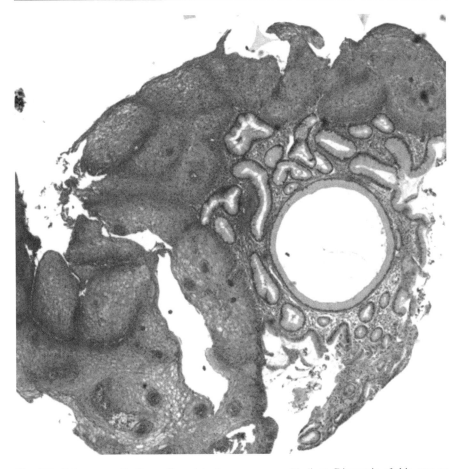

Fig. 5.2 Columnar epithelium adjacent to the squamous epithelium. Diagnosis of this case as Barrett's esophagus should depend upon the endoscopic findings as well as the histopathology. While pathologists from the USA require goblet cells for a definitive diagnosis, for European pathologists, columnar epithelium is sufficient for a diagnosis of Barrett's esophagus (H&E, original magnification ×10)

ESCC3: No deregulation of cell cycle was identified. PI3K pathway activation and somatic alterations in KMT2D/MLL2 and SMARCA4 were frequent, and these findings were not similar to those identified in head and neck SCC.

As expected, the molecular changes of the EAC cases were different from the ESCC cases, and they had similarities with the molecular changes observed in gastric carcinomas. The gastric carcinoma cases were grouped into four types according to the molecular findings: EBV-related, microsatellite instability, chromosomal instability, and genomic stability groups (Riquelme et al. 2015). The cases located at the esophagus rather than the gastric region were nearly consistent and had

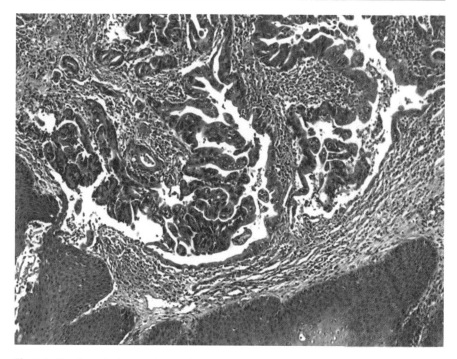

Fig. 5.3 Esophageal adenocarcinoma; note gland formation with tubulopapillary growth pattern typical for the carcinomas of this region (H&E, original magnification ×20)

features like the chromosomal instability group. DNA hypermethylation was more frequent in AEG junction cases compared to gastric chromosomal instability cases, and ERBB2, VEGFA, GATA4, and GATA6 were more commonly amplified in adenocarcinomas.

Prognostic Factors in Esophageal Carcinomas

ESCC and adenocarcinomas have differences in many aspects. In the series by Metzger et al. (2009), ESCC and adenocarcinoma cases were compared with special emphasis on perinodal invasion. Median survival for patients with extracapsular spread was shorter (13 months versus 28 months). Perinodal invasion was more frequent in metastatic adenocarcinoma cases compared with ESCC cases (66% versus 35%). The authors concluded that perinodal invasion was a poor prognostic feature more frequently observed in adenocarcinoma cases. Independent poor prognostic factors for esophageal carcinomas in this series included older age and high pT, pN, and pM categories as well as perinodal invasion.

Wang et al. (2017) evaluated a series of 446 ESCC cases, and of these 36.8% had lymph node metastasis. Larger tumor size, higher T stage, perineural invasion, and lymph node metastasis were independent prognostic factors in multivariate analysis. In a meta-analysis of 13 studies by Gao et al. (2016), perineural invasion was identified as a poor prognostic factor for disease-free and overall survival with hazard ratios of 1.96 and 1.76, respectively.

Lagarde et al. (2015) evaluated 396 esophageal carcinoma cases including ESCC and adenocarcinoma cases which received neoadjuvant therapy and focused on perineural, vascular, and lymphatic invasion. If three, two, one, and none of these factors were positive, the overall survival of the patients was 16, 27.1, 44.0, and 170.8 months, respectively. At the multivariate analysis, gender (female), adenocarcinoma histology, R0 resection, ypN, and the abovementioned findings (perineural, vascular, and lymphatic invasion) were identified as poor prognostic markers.

Proposed Mechanisms and Morphology of Tumor Deposits in Esophageal Carcinomas

There are very few studies about the tumor deposits (TDs) in esophageal carcinomas, and none of these proposed specific mechanisms for TD development. The morphology of the tumor deposits is not described in detail.

Classifications of Tumor Deposits in Esophageal Carcinomas

The only series about the tumor deposits in esophageal carcinomas is about adenocarcinoma cases at the gastroesophageal junction (Zhang HD); however, the authors did not present the criteria they applied in order to describe the lesions as tumor deposits. The images they presented do not have any lymph node structure or encapsulation which seems to be consistent with tumor deposits elsewhere; however, as the diagnostic criteria are not strictly described, we will also name them as extranodal metastasis (EM). Furthermore, at the discussion of the article, an article by Tanabe et al. (2007) referred to the same type of lesions as the squamous cell carcinomas of the esophagus. The lesions at the article by Tanabe et al. (2007) are consistent with perinodal invasion at the metastasis lymph nodes, making all the results of the article by Zhang et al. controversial (2013). One previous report in 2003 about the distal esophagus and gastroesophageal lymph nodes was about extracapsular lymph node involvement, and it seems the authors evaluated the impact of perinodal invasion on prognosis (Lerut et al. 2003).

Prognostic Studies on Tumor Deposits in Esophageal Carcinomas

In the series by Zhang et al. (2013), 284 patients with lymph node metastasis were evaluated. Among these cases, they found EM in 70 (24.6%) of the cases. EM was more frequent in large, undifferentiated, high-T-stage tumors and in cases with more metastatic lymph nodes. During the follow-up, 35% versus 60% of the patients without and with TD had recurrences ($p < 0.0001$). Cases with TD had peritoneal recurrences twice as frequently as the cases without TD (24.3% versus 12.1%, $p = 0.014$), but there was no statistically significant difference between hematogenous and local recurrence. EM-positive cases had shorter time till recurrence and experienced more recurrences compared to the EM-negative cases (16 months versus 36 months and 27.1% versus 7.1%). The positivity of EM increased the risk of recurrence by 2.786 times. Only 7.2% of EM-positive cases versus 29.9% of EM-negative cases were alive at 5 years, and the median survival time was 23 and 41 months. The EM positivity increased the risk of death by 2.159 times.

The independent prognostic factors for recurrence-free survival by multivariate analysis were depth of tumor invasion, N stage, and EM. For overall survival, the independent prognostic factors included depth of tumor invasion, N stage, and EM as poor prognostic markers and lymphadenectomy as a better prognostic marker.

Furthermore, the authors analyzed the survival of the patients after recurrence, who received second-line chemotherapy. The median time of survival for patients with EM was 4 months, while EM-negative cases survived for 8 months ($p = 0.035$).

Discussion About Tumor Deposits in Esophageal Carcinomas

The information about the TDs in esophageal carcinomas is rather sparse and would be an excellent research area. The lesions reflecting perinodal invasion and free TDs should be strictly defined and separated in any condition. The few previous reports that may be related to these lesions (Lerut T et al. 2003; Tanabe T et al. 2007; Zhang et al. 2013), "TDs," do not give histopathological criteria for diagnosis obscuring the results. The series best matching TDs was presented by Zhang et al. (2013), evaluating the incidence and prognostic value of TDs in AEG junction carcinomas, and their results were like the results achieved for gastric carcinomas (Chen et al. 2016; Ersen et al. 2014; Etoh et al. 2006; Jiang et al. 2014; Lee et al. 2013; Sun et al. 2012; Wang et al. 2011; Yildiz et al. 2016). In all the series, TDs were identified as poor prognostic markers. It is not unexpected that AEG junction adenocarcinomas have similar features with gastric adenocarcinomas. However, we don't have information about the ESCC in terms of TDs and their prognostic implications.

References

Cancer Genome Atlas Network. Comprehensive genomic characterization of head and neck squamous cell carcinomas. Nature. 2015;517:576–82.
Cancer Genome Atlas Research Network; Analysis Working Group. Integrated genomic characterization of oesophageal carcinoma. Nature. 2017;541(7636):169–75. https://doi.org/10.1038/nature20805. Epub 2017 Jan 4.
Cavallin F, Scarpa M, Alfieri R, Cagol M, Ruol A, Rugge M, Ancona E, Castoro C. Esophageal carcinosarcoma: management and prognosis at a single Italian series. Anticancer Res. 2014;34(12):7455–9.
Chen XL, Zhao LY, Xue L, Xu YH, Zhang WH, Liu K, Chen XZ, Yang K, Zhang B, Chen ZX, Chen JP, Zhou ZG, Hu JK. Prognostic significance and the role in TNM stage of

extranodal metastasis within regional lymph nodes station in gastric carcinoma. Oncotarget. 2016;7(41):67047–60. 10.18632/oncotarget.11478.

Ellis A, Risk JM, Maruthappu T, Kelsell DP. Tylosis with oesophageal cancer: diagnosis, management and molecular mechanisms. Orphanet J Rare Dis. 2015;10:126. https://doi.org/10.1186/s13023-015-0346-2.

Ersen A, Unlu MS, Akman T, Sagol O, Oztop I, Atila K, Bora S, Ellidokuz H, Sarioglu S. Tumor deposits in gastric carcinomas. Pathol Res Pract. 2014;210(9):565–70. https://doi.org/10.1016/j.prp.2014.03.006.

Etoh T, Sasako M, Ishikawa K, Katai H, Sano T, Shimoda T. Extranodal metastasis is an indicator of poor prognosis in patients with gastric carcinoma. Br J Surg. 2006;93(3):369–73.

Gao A, Wang L, Li J, Li H, Han Y, Ma X, Sun Y. Prognostic value of Perineural invasion in esophageal and esophagogastric junction carcinoma: a meta-analysis. Dis Markers. 2016;2016:7340180. https://doi.org/10.1155/2016/7340180.

https://seer.cancer.gov/statfacts/html/esoph.html. Accessed 12 July 2017.

Jain S, Dhingra S. Pathology of esophageal cancer and Barrett's esophagus. Ann Cardiothorac Surg. 2017;6(2):99–109. 10.21037/acs.2017.03.06.

Jiang N, Deng JY, Ding XW, Ke B, Liu N, Liang H. Node-extranodal soft tissue stage based on extranodal metastasis is associated with poor prognosis of patients with gastric cancer. J Surg Res. 2014;192(1):90–7. https://doi.org/10.1016/j.jss.2014.05.053.

Lagarde SM, Phillips AW, Navidi M, Disep B, Immanuel A, Griffin SM. The presence of lymphovascular and perineural infiltration after neoadjuvant therapy and oesophagectomy identifies patients at high risk for recurrence. Br J Cancer. 2015;113(10):1427–33. https://doi.org/10.1038/bjc.2015.354.

Lee HS, Lee HE, Yang HK, Kim WH. Perigastric tumor deposits in primary gastric cancer: implications for patient prognosis and staging. Ann Surg Oncol. 2013;20(5):1604–13. https://doi.org/10.1245/s10434-012-2692-9.

Lerut T, Coosemans W, Decker G, De Leyn P, Ectors N, Fieuws S, Moons J, Nafteux P, Van Raemdonck D, Leuven Collaborative Workgroup for Esophageal Carcinoma. Extracapsular lymph node involvement is a negative prognostic factor in T3 adenocarcinoma of the distal esophagus and gastroesophageal junction. J Thorac Cardiovasc Surg. 2003;126(4):1121–8.

Metzger R, Drebber U, Baldus SE, Mönig SP, Hölscher AH, Bollschweiler E. Extracapsular lymph node involvement differs between squamous cell and adenocarcinoma of the esophagus. Ann Surg Oncol. 2009;16(2):447–53.

O'Neill OM, Johnston BT, Coleman HG. Achalasia: a review of clinical diagnosis, epidemiology, treatment and outcomes. World J Gastroenterol. 2013;19(35):5806–12. https://doi.org/10.3748/wjg.v19.i35.5806.

Riquelme I, Saavedra K, Espinoza JA, Weber H, García P, Nervi B, Garrido M, Corvalán AH, Roa JC, Bizama C. Molecular classification of gastric cancer: towards a pathway-driven targeted therapy. Oncotarget. 2015;6(28):24750–79. 10.18632/oncotarget.4990.

Sun Z, Wang ZN, YY X, Zhu GL, Huang BJ, Xu Y, Liu FN, Zhu Z, Xu HM. Prognostic significance of tumor deposits in gastric cancer patients who underwent radical surgery. Surgery. 2012;151(6):871–81. https://doi.org/10.1016/j.surg.2011.12.027.

Tanabe T, Kanda T, Kosugi S, et al. Extranodal spreading of esophageal squamous cell carcinoma: clinicopathological characteristics and prognostic impact. World J Surg. 2007;31:2192–8.

Wang W, Li Y, Zhang Y, Yuan X, Xu D, Guan Y, Feng X, Chen Y, Sun X, Li W, Zhan Y, Zhou Z. Incorporation of extranodal metastasis of gastric carcinoma into the 7th edition UICC TNM staging system. PLoS One. 2011;6(6):e19557. https://doi.org/10.1371/journal.pone.0019557.

Wang H, Deng F, Liu Q, Ma Y. Prognostic significance of lymph node metastasis in esophageal squamous cell carcinoma. Pathol Res Pract. 2017;213(7):842–7. https://doi.org/10.1016/j.prp.2017.01.023.

Yildiz B, Etiz D, Dal P, Junushova B, Pasaoglu O, Yilmaz E, Erkasap S, Dincer M. Tumor deposits: prognostic significance in gastric cancer patients. J BUON. 2016;21(6):1476–81.

Zhang HD, Tang P, Duan XF, Chen CG, Ma Z, Gao YY, Zhang H, Yu ZT. Extranodal metastasis is a powerful prognostic factor in patients with adenocarcinoma of the esophagogastric junction. J Surg Oncol. 2013;108(8):542–9. https://doi.org/10.1002/jso.23430.

Peritoneal Carcinomatosis: Relation to Tumor Deposits

6

Peritoneal carcinomatosis may be caused by different types of carcinomas and tumors arising from different organs. Primary tumors of the peritoneum, like malignant mesothelioma, may result in this condition as well as different tumors metastatic to this region. This results in a complex area for diagnosis and treatment, which leads to information that is beyond the scope covered in this chapter. The possible mechanisms of peritoneal metastasis will be discussed along with some options of treatment.

Classification of the Peritoneal Carcinomatosis

Peritoneal carcinomatosis may be classified with different methods clinically and may be proven histopathologically if cytoreductive surgery is performed. The extent of the disease serves as a prognostic marker. The cases were classified into four stages by Gilly et al. (1999):

- Stage I: Malignant tumor nodules less than 5 mm in diameter localized in one part of the abdomen
- Stage II: Malignant tumor nodules less than 5 mm, diffuse to the whole abdomen
- Stage III: Tumor nodules of 5 mm to 2 cm diameter
- Stage IV: Large tumor deposits

Peritoneal carcinomatosis index (PCI) was proposed by Jacquet P and Sugarbaker PH in 1996 and has been used extensively afterward. In this scoring system, the abdomen is divided into 13 regions as follows: central, right upper, epigastric, left upper, left flank, left lower, pelvis, right upper, right flank, upper jejunum, lower jejunum, upper ileum, and lower ileum. The largest lesion at a region was scored as the "lesion size score" according to the criteria listed below:

© Springer International Publishing AG 2018

S. Sarioglu, *Tumor Deposits*, https://doi.org/10.1007/978-3-319-68582-3_6

- LS 0: No tumor seen
- LS 1: Tumor up to 0.5 cm
- LS 2: Tumor up to 5 cm
- LS 3: Tumor more than 5 cm

In this scoring system, each region is given a score according to "lesion size score," and addition of all these values for each region gives a peritoneal carcinomatosis score, ranging from 0 to 39. Different cut points have been given for these classification scores like "13" or "20" for statistical purposes, to find limited and extensive peritoneal carcinomatosis cases (Glehen et al. 2004; da Silva and Sugerbaker 2006).

Current treatment options of the peritoneal carcinomatosis include cytoreductive surgery and intraperitoneal hyperthermic chemotherapy. The completeness of the cytoreductive surgery (CCR) is related to the extent of the disease, and it is also an important prognostic marker. The score is given by the surgeon after the operation, and it is a strong predictor of prognosis that depends upon the criteria listed below:

- CCR-0: No macroscopic residual cancer remained.
- CCR-1: No residual nodule greater than 5 mm in diameter remained.
- CCR-2: Residual nodules greater than 5 mm (Glehen et al. 2004).

A preoperative scoring system for peritoneal malignancies was introduced by the American Society of Peritoneal Surface Malignancies that included symptoms of the patients, PCI index at the computed tomography scan, and histology of the primary tumor with good prognostic prediction (Esquivel et al. 2014).

Another approach may result in a classification of cases according to the distribution of tumoral lesions at the abdominal cavity, and this classification is as follows (Coccolini et al. 2013):

1. *Random proximal distribution (RPD)*: Early peritoneal implantation of moderate- and high-grade tumors like gastric and colorectal carcinomas and serous ovarian cancer, due to the adherence molecules on the surfaces of the cancer cells.
2. *Complete redistribution (CRD)*: The type that is typical for the cases with pseudomyxoma peritonei; adhesion of the peritoneal surfaces is not expected due to the low biological aggressiveness.
3. *Widespread cancer distribution (WCD)*: In these cases, the great amounts of mucinous material produced by some high-grade tumors, like grade II and III adenocarcinomas of the appendix and mucinous colorectal, gastric, or ovarian carcinomas, interfere with the activities of adhesion molecules.

Prognostic Factors in Peritoneal Carcinomatosis

Different types of tumors may result in peritoneal carcinomatosis. These include peritoneal mesothelioma, primary peritoneal carcinoma, pseudomyxoma peritonei which arises from the appendix in most of the cases, and gastric, ovarian, and colorectal carcinoma (Coccolini et al. 2013). Cytoreductive surgery and intraperitoneal chemotherapy improved the prognosis of peritoneal carcinoma cases without distant metastasis, other than resectable metastatic liver disease. The prognosis of peritoneal carcinoma cases is related to many factors including the primary tumor location, tumor type, extent of the disease, and treatment methods.

Different histopathological types and different primary tumor locations of carcinomas of the colorectum seem to have different types of metastatic potential. In an autopsy study of 1675 colorectal carcinoma patients by Hugen et al. (2014), mucinous and signet-ring carcinomas had metastasis and metastatic lesions at multiple sites more frequently than adenocarcinomas (33.9% and 61.2% versus 27.6% and 58.6% and 70.7% versus 49.9%, respectively). Most frequent metastatic sites were the lung and liver. Adenocarcinoma cases predominantly metastasized to the liver, and mucinous and signet-ring cell carcinomas metastasized to the peritoneum. Intra-abdominal metastasis was more frequent in colon carcinomas, and extra-abdominal metastasis was more frequent in rectal carcinoma cases.

Histopathological response to the preoperative chemotherapy was proposed as a prognostic marker in peritoneal carcinomatosis cases. Passot et al. (2014) evaluated the pathological response considering the viable cells in tumor nodules from each region, and three groups were created for statistical analysis: complete response, no cancer cells; major response, 1–49% residual cancer cells; and minor or no response, less than 50% residual cancer cells. For patients with multiple specimens, the mean of the values was used. Pathological response and FOLFOX therapy were the only independent prognostic markers in this series of cases treated by cytoreductive surgery and/or intraperitoneal chemotherapy. Minor and no pathological response increased the risk of death by 13.46 times and major response by 4.91 times.

Glehen et al. (2004) evaluated prognostic factors in a series of 506 patients from 28 institutions. The median survival of patients treated with complete cytoreductive surgery was 32.4 months, and this was 8.4 months for the patients who could not be operated with complete cytoreductive surgery. Positive independent prognostic factors were CCR0, treatment by a second operation, PCI score less than 13, younger age than 65, and the use of adjuvant chemotherapy. Negative independent prognostic factors were neoadjuvant chemotherapy, lymph node and liver metastasis, and poor differentiation.

In a series of 156 patients with peritoneal carcinomatosis arising from colorectal cancers, at the multivariate analysis, only PCI over 20 and metastatic lymph nodes were identified as poor prognostic markers (da Silva and Sugarbaker 2006). Prognosis of appendiceal mucinous neoplasms with peritoneal dissemination was found to be related to histological tumor type (hazard ratio = 3.13), high PCI index (>20), CRC score $\geq$ 2, early postoperative intraperitoneal chemotherapy, and CEA, CA19-9, and CA125 levels (Huang et al. 2017). Patients with gastric carcinomas and peritoneal carcinomatosis also seem to benefit from cytoreductive surgery and HIPEC increasing the survival nearly by two times (6.5–7 months versus 11–15 months). Results of few series about small bowel tumors with peritoneal carcinomatosis are consistent with improved survival with this type of therapy (Coccolini et al. 2013; Terzi et al. 2014).

In any case, PC cases should better be evaluated regarding the origin of the primary tumor. Appendiceal, colorectal, and gastric adenocarcinoma cases have different features related to prognosis following different types of treatment (Coccolini et al. 2013, Terzi et al. 2014).

Proposed Mechanisms of Neoplastic Lesions in Peritoneal Carcinomatosis

There are different theories about the mechanisms leading to peritoneal carcinomatosis. The most favored one is by shedding from the visceral peritoneum to the peritoneal cavity followed by attachment to different peritoneal and intraabdominal sites. This mechanism is the most widely accepted one; however, aside from this mechanism, lymph node metastasis and mechanisms leading to tumor deposit formation may also have some contribution.

Visceral Peritoneal Invasion, Spillage to the Peritoneal Cavity, and Seeding

It was suggested by Koppe et al. (2014) that the spread from the gastrointestinal tract to the peritoneum may take place at different times:

- In cases with visceral peritoneal invasion, there may be spillage at the preoperative stage.
- Rupture of the organ by the obstruction caused by the tumor or other reasons.
- Spillage of the tumor cells during operation.

Shelygin et al. (2014) compared the genetical changes in colorectal carcinomas with and without peritoneal metastasis. They compared the expression of genes, which may be accepted as markers of epithelial-mesenchymal transition (*ZEB1, ZEB2, CDH1, VIM,* and *SNAI1* expression and *CDH1* downregulation), *KRAS* and *BRAF* mutations, and microsatellite instability status, in a series of 58 cases, of which 20 had peritoneal metastasis. Expression patterns reflecting epithelial-mesenchymal transition were identified in 15.79% of the cases without peritoneal metastasis, 35% of the cases with peritoneal metastasis, and 95% of peritoneal metastatic nodules. High histopathological grade, *KRAS* mutation, and *BRAF*V600E mutations were more frequent in cases with peritoneal carcinomatosis and in cases with expression patterns consistent with epithelial-mesenchymal transition phenotype, but there was no difference when microsatellite instability was considered. There are additional studies showing the association of epithelial-mesenchymal transition with *KRAS* mutations at G12V and *BRAF*V600E mutations in colorectal carcinoma cases (Makrodouli et al. 2011).

Separation of the carcinoma cells from the visceral peritoneal surfaces of the abdominal organs and seeding at the peritoneal surfaces followed by invasion of the carcinoma cells to the peritoneal surfaces seem to be a very important mechanism of metastasis and tumor recurrence. In a review about the role of mesothelial cells in peritoneal dissemination, Rynne-Vidal et al. (2015) reported the peritoneal cavity as the site of metastases in up to 28% endometrial, 42% of colorectal, 40% of gastric, and 70% of ovarian recurrent carcinomas. The "seed and soil" hypothesis proposed by Stephan Paget in 1899 is more alive than ever and has increasing value in oncological studies as tumor-associated fibroblasts are very important in the survival of the seed (Paget 1989). At the peritoneal metastasis, for "seeding," the mesothelial cells seem to play important roles.

A set of cells may transform into the myofibroblasts or cancer-associated fibroblasts (CAFs) including resident fibroblasts, bone marrow-derived stem cells, endothelial cells, and mesothelial cells as well as cancer cells. The origin of CAFs from mesothelial cells was highlighted with immunohistochemistry by showing calretinin, WT1, and mesothelin expression, the markers of mesothelial differentiation, in cells surrounding neoplastic cells, deeply invasive away from the peritoneal surfaces. The steps during transition of mesothelial cells to CAFs include decreasing of intercellular adhesion molecules, loss of microvilli and apicobasal polarity, α-smooth muscle actin expression, and basement membrane degradation leading to migratory capacity. The malignant ascites fluid may contribute to this transition as it is very rich in many types of cytokines and growth factors including TNF-β1, a prototypical inducer of epithelial-mesenchymal transition originating from the malignant cells (Thibault et al. 2014). Furthermore exosomes are also important in the transfer of these soluble factors including proteins and miRNAs from the neoplastic cells to the mesothelial cells (Vaksman et al. 2014).

The possible mechanisms of peritoneal attachment by the neoplastic cells were evaluated (Kusamura et al. 2010). Adhesion to the mesothelial cells or connective tissues was proposed as an alternative. The mesothelial cells with features of mesenchymal transition promote invasive properties of the carcinoma cells. Satoyoshi et al. (2015) suggested that mesothelial cells with invasive properties act as a leading front for the carcinoma cell invasion to the deep layers of peritoneum through Tks5 activation. During this process, the matrix metalloproteinases (MMPs) and their inhibitors are important like in chemical peritoneal fibrosis models (Borazan et al. 2009). These findings led to the co-invasion hypothesis of the neoplastic cells and mesothelial cells leading to peritoneal metastasis, which should follow the steps described above, like TGF-β1 induction of the mesothelial cells or the exosome-transported information to the mesothelial cells for mesenchymal transition and β1 integrin-related adhesion. For the peritoneal metastasis to produce a mass that may be detected clinically, it is not hard to guess the necessity of tumor cell proliferation and angiogenesis as well as extracellular matrix remodeling with the contribution of the mesothelial-derived CAFs secreting vascular endothelial growth factor, MMPs, fibronectin, collagen, etc. (Rynne-Vidal et al. 2015).

Omentum and Milky Spots

"Milky spots" (MS) are sites of peritoneal colonization. They are unique secondary lymphoid organs recognized by capillaries surrounded by immune cells (Rangel-Moreno et al. 2009; Liu et al. 2015). These areas are best targets for metastatic cell colonization and CAFs accumulate at these sites. They were described by Recklinghausen in rabbits in 1863, and after 130 years, they were recognized as main sites of implantation and dissemination.

The most frequent site for MS is the omentum; however, they are also found in the gonadal fat, mesenterium, posterior abdominal wall, stomach, liver, intestine, anterior abdominal wall, and lung in decreasing quantities; the pleura is also another site (Hagiwara et al. 1993).

The MS are rich in T lymphocytes, followed by B lymphocytes and macrophages (46.1%, 28.4%, and 12.4%, respectively), lacking dendritic cells. They may be oval, round, or irregularly shaped with a mean diameter of 140.2 (41.6–395.1) μm. (Rynne-Vidal et al. 2015). MS act as macrophage maturation sites during gestation (Liu et al. 2015). MS are important in defense against cancer cells with the cytotoxic T cells, and also they act as a filter; however, this increases the risk of being a metastatic site in a person with a malignant tumor. Tumor-associated macrophages (TAMs) may act against the tumor cells or help the cancer cells in angiogenesis, invasion, and proliferation, if they are in a cancer cell remodeled stage (Liu et al. 2013). TAMs, CAFs, and mesothelial cells with mesenchymal transition serve the cancer cells during the steps of peritoneal carcinogenesis.

There are hypoxic areas at the milky spots that may be observed with hypoxia-inducible factor-1 α expression, leading to increased number of tumor cells with stem cell phenotype and aggressive tumor clones, while the stem cells of the fat tissue may support the tumor growth; adipocytes provide fatty acids for growth of the cancer cells as well as promoting homing, migration, and invasion (Koppe et al. 2014; Rynne-Vidal et al. 2015).

Treatment Options

The options of cytoreductive surgery and intraperitoneal chemotherapy have influenced the grave prognosis of the patients with peritoneal carcinomatosis; however, options for prevention are always better than treatments following recurrences. Although the complications related to these treatment modalities may be in an acceptable range, they still exist (Sugarbaker 2014; Canda et al. 2013). Understanding the mechanisms underlying peritoneal implantation and invasion in relation with changes of the mesothelial cells has led the researchers to therapeutic options which might prevent the development of peritoneal carcinomatoses, targeting the mesothelial cell changes. Blockage of TGF-β1 was proven to be effective in both in vitro and in vivo studies in preventing peritoneal dissemination (Miao et al. 2014). Bone morphogenetic protein-7 is known to reduce or reverse mesenchymal transition of the mesothelial cells and may be a useful option. The inhibition of inflammation may be a method for saving the peritoneal surface integrity. Effect of cyclooxygenase (COX)-2 inhibitors was evaluated in different settings like in peritoneal rat endometriosis model (Dogan et al. 2004). COX-2 expression is increased in different types of carcinomas leading to increased mesenchymal transition of the mesothelial cells, and the blockage may be beneficial for inhibiting mesenchymal transition of the mesothelial cells (Midgley et al. 2010). Blockage of the mesothelial cell adhesion molecules, inhibitors of MMPs, and tamoxifen as a preservative of mesothelial cells and blockage of vascular endothelial growth factor and/or its receptors might be alternatives (Rynne-Vidal et al. 2015).

Whether it is beneficial for the patients to remove the omentum in early stages of cancer progression is a subject of debate as the experimental studies are in favor of the omentum's role in preventing peritoneal carcinomatosis in these settings. Even at the later stages, the results are inconclusive if there is no evidence of macroscopic disease (Koppe et al. 2014).

Lymphatic Route

The extensive evidence and studies in peritoneal carcinomatosis are centered at the dissemination from the late-stage gastrointestinal carcinomas through the peritoneal surfaces as described above. However, some cases with abdominal malignancies, without invasion to the peritoneal surfaces, may present with peritoneal carcinomatosis, leading to the search for possibilities of different mechanisms. Yamamoto et al. (2006) presented an early gastric carcinoma case with positive peritoneal cytology and reviewed the literature and found 15 cases with peritoneal carcinomatosis of early gastric cancer. Early-stage gastrointestinal carcinomas with peritoneal carcinomatosis may be evidence in favor of other routes from peritoneal dissemination. Yoshida et al. (2016) presented five early gastric carcinoma patients with peritoneal carcinomatosis in a series of 1509 cases. Although there are very few cases like this, they are valuable for providing evidence about other routes of dissemination. Peritoneal carcinomatosis is a feature of disease of late stages in most of the cases, at which time invasion of visceral peritoneum and blood and lymphatic vessels is frequent and specification of the mechanism at this point is difficult. The early carcinoma cases provide evidence that transmural invasion is not the only mechanism for dissemination. Yoshida et al. proposed that the mechanism might be, submucosal lymphatic invasion, transfer to the lymphatics at the serosa and/or regional lymph nodes and dissemination to the peritoneum. Shedding from metastatic lymph nodes or lymphatic channels might be another explanation. Of the five cases in the series of Yoshida et al. (2016), two cases had many metastatic lymph nodes as well as tumor deposits, and both were dead in 3 and 16 months. The authors found lymphatic invasion in all cases and vascular invasion in one case, but there was no information about the perineural invasion.

Tumor Deposits and Peritoneal Carcinomatosis

Etoh et al. (2006), Zhang et al. (2013), and Jiang et al. (2014) showed the frequent association of tumor deposits with peritoneal carcinomatosis in gastric and esophagogastric junction carcinoma cases. In the series of Etoh et al. (2006), 146 patients had tumor deposits among 1023 cases of gastric carcinomas. The cases with tumor deposits had peritoneal metastasis in 40.4% of the cases, while the cases without tumor deposits had peritoneal carcinomatosis in only 2.3% of the cases. The prognostic studies in this series showed similar poor prognosis in cases with tumor deposits and peritoneal carcinomatosis. In the series of Zhang et al. (2013), 284 gastroesophageal junction adenocarcinoma cases were evaluated, and in 24.6% of the cases, there were tumor deposits. The rate of peritoneal recurrence between patients with and without tumor deposits was significantly different (24.3% and 12.1%, respectively). The authors suggested that tumor deposits might be included in M category like peritoneal carcinomatosis. In the series by Jiang et al. (2014), 642 gastric carcinoma patients were evaluated, and tumor deposits were identified in 26.79% of the cases. Tumor deposits were found as the highest risk factor for peritoneal recurrence with a 2.448 odds ratio. Peritoneal recurrence was identified in 37.8% versus 17% of the cases with and without tumor deposits. The authors suggested that tumor deposits should be included in the M category of tumor staging considering the poor prognostic features and association with peritoneal metastasis.

These articles highlight the significant association between tumor deposits and peritoneal carcinomatosis; however, the mechanisms leading to this relation have not been explained yet. If lymphatic route is important in at least some of the cases, mechanisms leading to tumor deposit formation may also be an important mechanism.

Morphology of Tumoral Lesions in Peritoneal Carcinomatosis

The morphological features of tumoral lesions may be different in peritoneal carcinomatosis. In some cases, different morphological features may be observed in a single patient.

The superficial tumor nodules connected to the peritoneal surface are easily identified as nodules formed by shedding and seeding of the tumor cells from the serosal surfaces (Figs. 6.1 and 6.2).

In some of the lesions, the connection with the surface (parietal peritoneum) cannot be observed; the neoplastic lesions may have smooth or irregular contours (Figs. 6.3, 6.4, and 6.5).

Peritoneal carcinomatosis or the tumoral involvement of the omental lesions does not always form nodular lesions, and sometimes diffuse lesions may be seen as in the examples from a poorly cohesive and signet-ring cell gastric carcinoma case (Figs. 6.6, 6.7, 6.8, and 6.9).

In some cases, there may be extensive lymphatic invasion, and these cases may be associated with formation of tumor nodules (Figs. 6.10 and 6.11). In some cases, tumor nodules resembling tumor deposits may be observed, and some of these may be located adjacent to vascular structures like the lesions observed in perivascular migratory metastasis (Figs. 6.12 and 6.13).

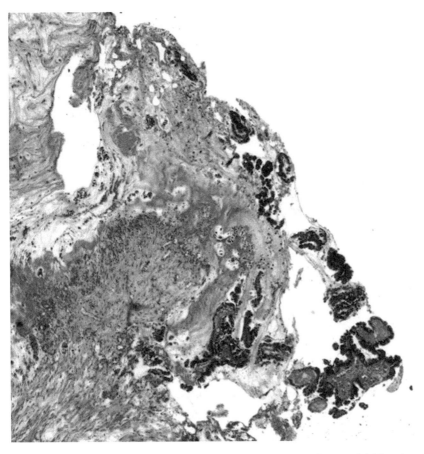

Fig. 6.1 Peritoneal carcinomatosis of a colon carcinoma case. Note the superficial location of the neoplastic lesion with inflammatory and fibrotic reaction (H&E, original magnification ×100)

Multiple metastatic lesions in patients with peritoneal carcinomatosis may be grouped as nodular and diffuse like in Figs. 6.1, 6.2, 6.3, 6.4, 6.5, 6.10, and 6.13, versus Figs. 6.6, 6.7, 6.8, 6.9, and 6.10 as well as in three types as follows:

- All tumoral deposits are in contact with the peritoneum.
- None of the nodules are connected to the peritoneum.
- A mixture of these two types.

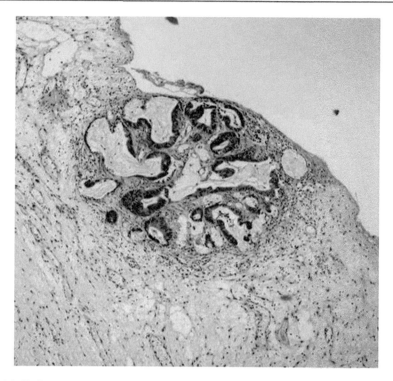

Fig. 6.2 Peritoneal carcinomatosis of a colon carcinoma case. Note the superficial location of the neoplastic lesion; the relation with the peritoneum is preserved (H&E, original magnification ×100)

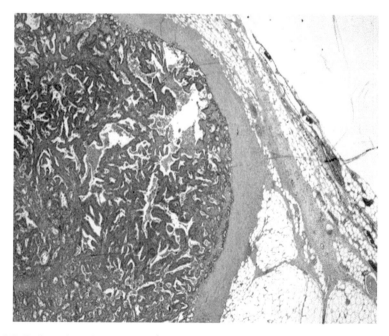

Fig. 6.3 Peritoneal carcinomatosis lesion arising from a colon carcinoma, separate from the mesothelial layer with a fibrotic capsule (H&E, original magnification ×100)

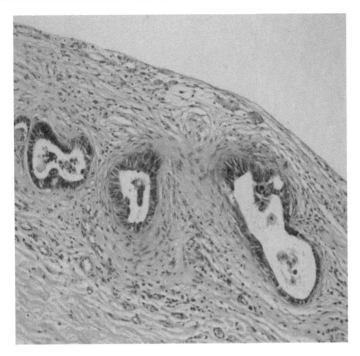

Fig. 6.4 Peritoneal carcinomatosis lesion arising from a colon carcinoma, separate from the mesothelial layer in a desmoplastic stroma (H&E, original magnification ×200)

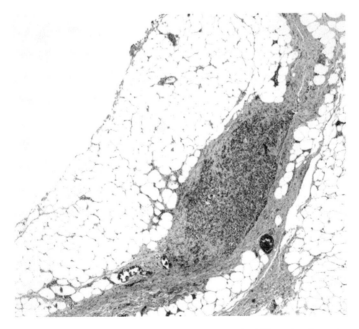

Fig. 6.5 Peritoneal carcinomatosis lesion arising from a poorly differentiated gastric carcinoma, separate from the mesothelial layer mimicking the morphology of milky spots, surrounded by some lymphocytes (H&E, original magnification ×40)

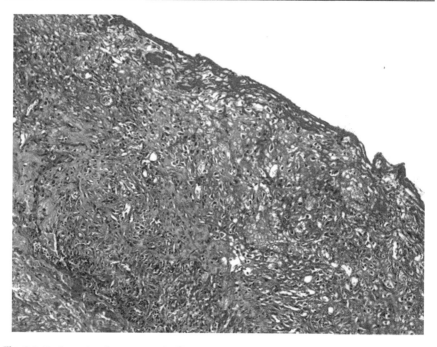

Fig. 6.6 Peritoneal surface covered by fibrin and diffuse carcinoma involvement of the underlying region with desmoplastic reaction (H&EX original magnification ×100)

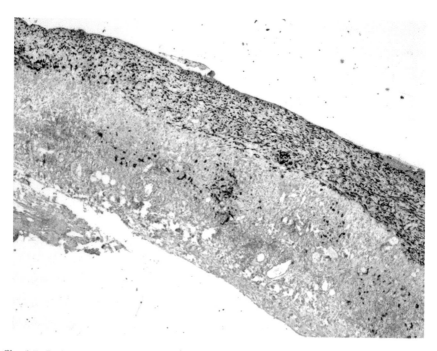

Fig. 6.7 Peritoneal surface covered by fibrin and diffuse carcinoma involvement of the underlying region with desmoplastic reaction (Pan-keratin, original magnification ×40)

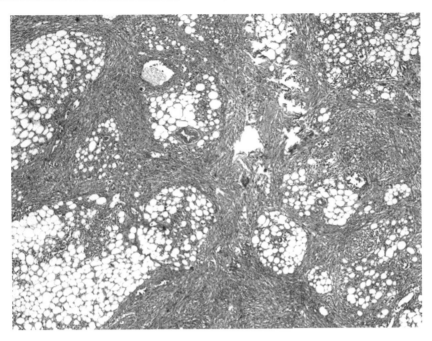

Fig. 6.8 Omentum with diffuse involvement with carcinoma surrounded by inflammation and desmoplastic reaction (H&EX original magnification ×100)

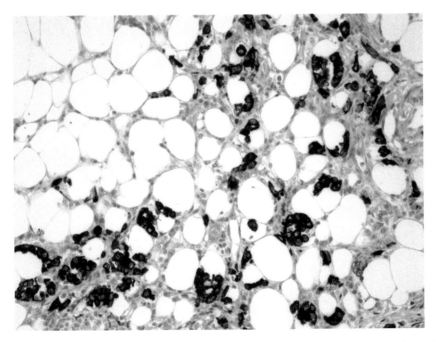

Fig. 6.9 Omentum with diffuse involvement with carcinoma surrounded by inflammation and desmoplastic reaction (Pan-keratin, original magnification ×400)

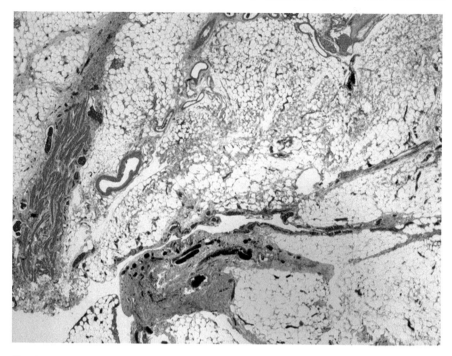

Fig. 6.10 Many lymphatics are filled with high-grade gastric carcinoma cells (H&EX original magnification ×100)

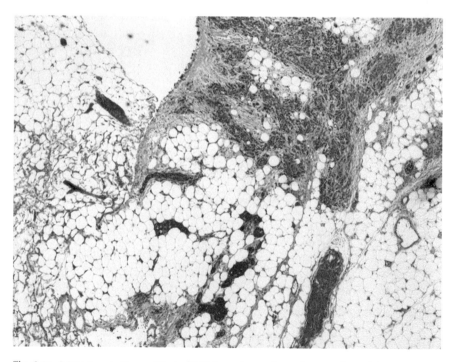

Fig. 6.11 Many lymphatics are filled with high-grade gastric carcinoma cells, and there is a tumor nodule adjacent to these lymphatics (H&EX original magnification ×100)

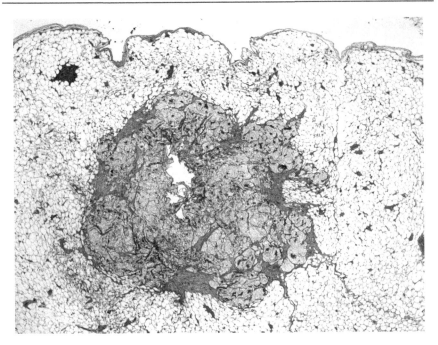

Fig. 6.12 Peritoneal carcinomatosis arising from mucinous carcinoma of the colon, morphologically not different from a tumor deposit at the colon serosa (H&EX original magnification ×100)

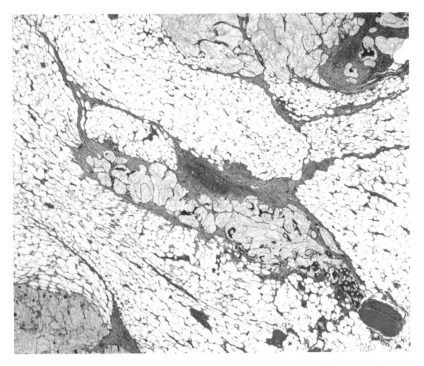

Fig. 6.13 Peritoneal carcinomatosis arising from mucinous carcinoma of the colon adjacent to a vascular structure, not different from a tumor deposit at the colon serosa which might have developed with the perivascular migratory invasion mechanism (H&EX original magnification ×100)

Discussion About Tumor Deposits in Peritoneal Carcinomatosis

The morphology of the peritoneal carcinomatosis cases resembles tumor deposits in a group of cases. Considering the small group of early gastric carcinoma cases with lymph node metastasis and peritoneal carcinomatosis, similar mechanisms might be questioned in relation with tumor deposits (Yoshida et al. 2016). The formation of tumor deposits by spillage from peritoneal surface, implantation, invasion with CAFs, and mesenchymal transferred mesothelial cells has been well studied, and many steps of the mechanisms have been explained. However, the mechanisms leading to tumor deposit formation might be related to mechanisms leading to peritoneal carcinomatosis at least in some of the cases with nodules that are not connected to the peritoneum; the increased peritoneal carcinomatosis lesions in cases with tumor deposits should not be overlooked (Etoh et al. 2006; Zhang et al. 2013, and Jiang et al. 2014). Some of the lesions in peritoneal carcinomatosis cases share many morphological features of tumor deposits elsewhere. However, the hypothesis in this context is not proven yet and this may be a research area.

The formation of tumor deposits in different parts of the body has not been explained like the peritoneal carcinomatosis cases mentioned above. Plaza et al. (2008) presented 118 cases metastatic to the soft tissues as tumor deposits, and the majority of the cases were metastases of carcinomas, followed by malignant melanoma, sarcoma, and others. Following this series, soft tissue tumor deposits have been presented in many reports, but mechanisms leading to this rare phenomenon were not clear other than the unproven possibility of hematogenous spread.

References

Borazan A, Camsari T, Cavdar Z, Sarioglu S, Yilmaz O, Oktay G, Sifil A, Celik A, Cavdar C, Aysal A, Kolatan E. The effects of darbepoetin on peritoneal fibrosis induced by chemical peritonitis and on peritoneal tissue MMP2 and TIMP-2 levels in rats. Eur J Inflamm. 2009;7(2): 87–95.

Canda AE, Sokmen S, Terzi C, Arslan C, Oztop I, Karabulut B, Ozzeybek D, Sarioglu S, Fuzun M. Complications and toxicities after cytoreductive surgery and hyperthermic intraperitoneal chemotherapy. Ann Surg Oncol. 2013;20(4):1082–7. https://doi.org/10.1245/s10434-012-2853-x; Epub 2013 Mar 2.

Coccolini F, Gheza F, Lotti M, Virzì S, Iusco D, Ghermandi C, Melotti R, Baiocchi G, Giulini SM, Ansaloni L, Catena F. Peritoneal carcinomatosis. World J Gastroenterol. 2013;19(41):6979–94. https://doi.org/10.3748/wjg.v19.i41.6979.

da Silva RG, Sugarbaker PH. Analysis of prognostic factors in seventy patients having a complete cytoreduction plus perioperative intraperitoneal chemotherapy for carcinomatosis from colorectal cancer. J Am Coll Surg. 2006;203(6):878–86.

Dogan E, Saygili U, Posaci C, Tuna B, Caliskan S, Altunyurt S, Saatli B. Regression of endometrial explants in rats treated with the cyclooxygenase-2 inhibitor rofecoxib. Fertil Steril. 2004;82(Suppl 3):1115–20.

Esquivel J, Lowy AM, Markman M, Chua T, Pelz J, Baratti D, Baumgartner JM, Berri R, Bretcha-Boix P, Deraco M, Flores-Ayala G, Glehen O, Gomez-Portilla A, González-Moreno S, Goodman M, Halkia E, Kusamura S, Moller M, Passot G, Pocard M, Salti G, Sardi A, Senthil M, Spilioitis J, Torres-Melero J, Turaga K, Trout R. The American Society of Peritoneal Surface Malignancies (ASPSM) Multiinstitution Evaluation of the Peritoneal Surface Disease Severity

Score (PSDSS) in 1,013 Patients with Colorectal Cancer with Peritoneal Carcinomatosis. Ann Surg Oncol. 2014;21(13):4195–201. https://doi.org/10.1245/s10434-014-3798-z; Epub 2014 May 23.

Etoh T, Sasako M, Ishikawa K, Katai H, Sano T, Shimoda T. Extranodal metastasis is an indicator of poor prognosis in patients with gastric carcinoma. Br J Surg. 2006;93(3):369–73.

Gilly FN, Beaujard A, Glehen O, Grandclement E, Caillot JL, Francois Y, Sadeghi-Looyeh B, Gueugniaud PY, Garbit F, Benoit M, Bienvenu J, Vignal J. Peritonectomy combined with intra-peritoneal chemohyperthermia in abdominal cancer with peritoneal carcinomatosis: phase I-II study. Anticancer Res. 1999;19(3B):2317–21.

Glehen O, Kwiatkowski F, Sugarbaker PH, Elias D, Levine EA, De Simone M, Barone R, Yonemura Y, Cavaliere F, Quenet F, Gutman M, Tentes AA, Lorimier G, Bernard JL, Bereder JM, Porcheron J, Gomez-Portilla A, Shen P, Deraco M, Rat P. Cytoreductive surgery combined with perioperative intraperitoneal chemotherapy for the management of peritoneal carcinoma-tosis from colorectal cancer: a multi-institutional study. J Clin Oncol. 2004;22(16):3284–92.

Hagiwara A, Takahashi T, Sawai K, Taniguchi H, Shimotsuma M, Okano S, Sakakura C, Tsujimoto H, Osaki K, Sasaki S, et al. Milky spots as the implantation site for malignant cells in peritoneal dissemination in mice. Cancer Res. 1993;53(3):687–92.

Huang Y, Alzahrani NA, Chua TC, Morris DL. Histological subtype remains a significant prog-nostic factor for survival outcomes in patients with appendiceal mucinous neoplasm with peritoneal dissemination. Dis Colon Rectum. 2017;60(4):360–7. https://doi.org/10.1097/DCR.0000000000000719.

Hugen N, van de Velde CJ, de Wilt JH, Nagtegaal ID. Metastatic pattern in colorectal cancer is strongly influenced by histological subtype. Ann Oncol. 2014;25(3):651–7. https://doi.org/10.1093/annonc/mdt591; Epub 2014 Feb 6.

Jacquet P, Sugarbaker PH. Clinical research methodologies in diagnosis and staging of patients with peritoneal carcinomatosis. Cancer Treat Res. 1996;82:359–74.

Jiang N, Deng JY, Ding XW, Ke B, Liu N, Liang H. Node-extranodal soft tissue stage based on extranodal metastasis is associated with poor prognosis of patients with gastric cancer. J Surg Res. 2014;192(1):90–7. https://doi.org/10.1016/j.jss.2014.05.053; Epub 2014 May 23.

Koppe MJ, Nagtegaal ID, de Wilt JH, Ceelen WP. Recent insights into the pathophysiology of omental metastases. J Surg Oncol. 2014;110(6):670–5. https://doi.org/10.1002/jso.23681; Epub 2014 Jun 24.

Kusamura S, Baratti D, Zaffaroni N, Villa R, Laterza B, Balestra MR, Deraco M. Pathophysiology and biology of peritoneal carcinomatosis. World J Gastrointest Oncol. 2010;2(1):12–8. https://doi.org/10.4251/wjgo.v2.i1.12.

Liu JY, Yuan JP, Geng XF, Qu AP, Li Y. Morphological study and comprehensive cellular con-stituents of milky spots in the human omentum. Int J Clin Exp Pathol. 2015;8(10):12877–84. eCollection 2015.

Liu XY, Miao ZF, Zhao TT, Wang ZN, Xu YY, Gao J, Wu JH, You Y, Xu H, Xu HM. Milky spot macrophages remodeled by gastric cancer cells promote peritoneal mesothelial cell injury. Biochem Biophys Res Commun. 2013;439(3):378–83. https://doi.org/10.1016/j.bbrc.2013.08.073; Epub 2013 Aug 29.

Makrodouli E, Oikonomou E, Koc M, Andera L, Sasazuki T, Shirasawa S, Pintzas A. BRAF and RAS oncogenes regulate Rho GTPase pathways to mediate migration and invasion properties in human colon cancer cells: a comparative study. Mol Cancer. 2011;10:118. https://doi.org/10.1186/1476-4598-10-118.

Miao ZF, Zhao TT, Wang ZN, Miao F, Xu YY, Mao XY, Gao J, Wu JH, Liu XY, You Y, Xu H, Xu HM. Transforming growth factor-beta1 signaling blockade attenuates gastric cancer cell-induced peritoneal mesothelial cell fibrosis and alleviates peritoneal dissemination both in vitro and in vivo. Tumour Biol. 2014;35(4):3575–83. https://doi.org/10.1007/s13277-013-1472-x; Epub 2013 Dec 18.

Midgley RS, McConkey CC, Johnstone EC, Dunn JA, Smith JL, Grumett SA, Julier P, Iveson C, Yanagisawa Y, Warren B, Langman MJ, Kerr DJ. Phase III randomized trial assessing rofe-coxib in the adjuvant setting of colorectal cancer: final results of the VICTOR trial. J Clin Oncol. 2010;28(30):4575–80. https://doi.org/10.1200/JCO.2010.29.6244; Epub 2010 Sep 13.

Paget S. The distribution of secondary growths in cancer of the breast. 1889. Cancer Metastasis Rev. 1989;8(2):98–101.

Passot G, You B, Boschetti G, Fontaine J, Isaac S, Decullier E, Maurice C, Vaudoyer D, Gilly FN, Cotte E, Glehen O. Pathological response to neoadjuvant chemotherapy: a new prognosis tool for the curative management of peritoneal colorectal carcinomatosis. Ann Surg Oncol. 2014;21(8):2608–14. https://doi.org/10.1245/s10434-014-3647-0; Epub 2014 Mar 26.

Plaza JA, Perez-Montiel D, Mayerson J, Morrison C, Suster S. Metastases to soft tissue: a review of 118 cases over a 30-year period. Cancer. 2008;112(1):193–203.

Rangel-Moreno J, Moyron-Quiroz JE, Carragher DM, Kusser K, Hartson L, Moquin A, et al. Omental milky spots develop in the absence of lymphoid tissue-inducer cells and support B and T cell responses to peritoneal antigens. Immunity. 2009;731–43(26):30.

Rynne-Vidal A, Jiménez-Heffernan JA, Fernández-Chacón C, López-Cabrera M, Sandoval P. The mesothelial origin of carcinoma associated-fibroblasts in peritoneal metastasis. Cancers (Basel). 2015;7(4):1994–2011. https://doi.org/10.3390/cancers7040872.

Satoyoshi R, Aiba N, Yanagihara K, Yashiro M, Tanaka M. Tks5 activation in mesothelial cells creates invasion front of peritoneal carcinomatosis. Oncogene. 2015;34(24):3176–87. https://doi.org/10.1038/onc.2014.246; Epub 2014 Aug 4.

Shelygin YA, Pospekhova NI, Shubin VP, Kashnikov VN, Frolov SA, Sushkov OI, Achkasov SI, Tsukanov AS. Epithelial-mesenchymal transition and somatic alteration in colorectal cancer with and without peritoneal carcinomatosis. Biomed Res Int. 2014;2014:629496. https://doi.org/10.1155/2014/629496; Epub 2014 Aug 3.

Sugarbaker HP. Update on the prevention of local recurrence and peritoneal metastases in patients with colorectal cancer. World J Gastroenterol. 2014;20(28):9286–91.

Terzi C, Arslan NC, Canda AE. Peritoneal carcinomatosis of gastrointestinal tumors: where are we now? World J Gastroenterol. 2014;20(39):14371–80. https://doi.org/10.3748/wjg.v20.i39.14371.

Thibault B, Castells M, Delord JP, Couderc B. Ovarian cancer microenvironment: implications for cancer dissemination and chemoresistance acquisition. Cancer Metastasis Rev. 2014;33(1):17–39. https://doi.org/10.1007/s10555-013-9456-2.

Vaksman O, Tropé C, Davidson B, Reich R. Exosome-derived miRNAs and ovarian carcinoma progression. Carcinogenesis. 2014;35(9):2113–20. https://doi.org/10.1093/carcin/bgu130; Epub 2014 Jun 12.

Yamamoto M, Taguchi K, Baba H, Endo K, Kohnoe S, Okamura T, Maehara Y. Peritoneal dissemination of early gastric cancer: report of a case. Surg Today. 2006;36(9):835–8.

Yoshida M, Sugino T, Kusafuka K, Nakajima T, Makuuchi R, Tokunaga M, Tanizawa Y, Bando E, Kawamura T, Terashima M, Kawata N, Tanaka M, Kakushima N, Takizawa K, Ono H. Peritoneal dissemination in early gastric cancer: importance of the lymphatic route. Virchows Arch. 2016;469(2):155–61. https://doi.org/10.1007/s00428-016-1960-7; Epub 2016 May 25.

Zhang HD, Tang P, Duan XF, Chen CG, Ma Z, Gao YY, Zhang H, Yu ZT. Extranodal metastasis is a powerful prognostic factor in patients with adenocarcinoma of the esophagogastric junction. J Surg Oncol. 2013;108(8):542–9. https://doi.org/10.1002/jso.23430; Epub 2013 Sep 9.

Tumor Deposits in Salivary Gland Carcinomas

7

Morphological diversity of salivary gland malignant tumors is remarkable. The behavior of malignant tumors may be different from favorable to poor. The histological structure of the major and minor salivary glands starts with acini emptying into intercalated ducts which are lined by myoepithelial cells helping the luminal movement of saliva following the route to larger ducts and finally to the oral cavity. Some of the neoplasms have features mimicking the histological features of the different parts of the gland. Salivary gland tumors do not only arise from major salivary glands (parotid, submandibular, and sublingual) and intraoral minor salivary glands, but they may arise from seromucinous glands of the respiratory tract. They may arise from the nasal cavity, paranasal sinuses, larynx, trachea, and lungs (Gibault and Badoual 2016), breast (Foschini et al. 2017), and thymus (Kalhor et al. 2017). More than 20 types of malignant tumors are included at the last World Health Organization classification in 2017, and histopathological classification of these tumors is a challenge for histopathologists (Etit et al. 2013).

Like in many types of malignant tumors, determining prognostic factors in salivary gland tumors is also very important. However, due to some specific features of the salivary gland tumors, it is hard to identify prognostic markers. Malignant salivary gland tumors are rare. They may arise from a wide spectrum of anatomical sites, and the sites may have prognostic significance. The diversity of the histopathological tumor types and changing classifications with inclusion of new and different types of carcinomas complicate the issue further. In spite of these, tumor and lymph node stage, age, sex, perineural invasion, facial palsy, histopathological type, grade, skin or bone invasion, extracapsular spread, margin status, and anatomical site were identified as poor prognostic markers either for disease-free or overall survival in large series (Terhaard et al. 2004; Walvekar et al. 2011; Carrillo et al. 2007).

Many prognostic factors important in different types of carcinomas have been evaluated in salivary gland tumors, but there is little information about the tumor deposits. Tumor deposits (TDs), which were described for the first time in colorectal carcinomas by Gabriel WB in 1935, have been identified as a poor prognostic factor in many series and in different types of carcinomas. TDs were included in the

© Springer International Publishing AG 2018
S. Sarioglu, *Tumor Deposits*, https://doi.org/10.1007/978-3-319-68582-3_7

colorectal TNM staging in 2009 in the 7th edition (Sobin 2009). According to the College of American Pathologists Cancer Protocols for colorectal carcinomas, the tumor deposits are described as "tumor nodules with regular or irregular contours, located away from the primary tumor mass, but within the lymphatic draining area, devoid of the morphological features of a lymph node," and such lesions exist also at the drainage area of the salivary gland tumors of neck dissection specimens in particular.

Histopathological Classification of Salivary Gland Malignant Tumors

Classification of the salivary gland tumors was revised in 2017. In each classification of the salivary gland tumors by the World Health Organization, new tumor types were included making the group of tumors named as *adenocarcinoma not otherwise specified* smaller. The recently added group of carcinomas in the last edition is based on both histopathological and molecular pathological features. Mammary analogue secretory carcinoma is the most important entity included in the last WHO classification (Seethala and Stenman 2017). A brief overview of the salivary gland malignant tumors is as follows:

– *Mucoepidermoid carcinoma:*
   This tumor is cystic or solid and made up of three types of cells: mucin-producing, intermediate, and squamoid. Translocation (11;19)(q21;p13) resulting in CRTC1-MALM2 gene fusion is frequent, and it is suggested that this type of translocation is seen especially in low-grade tumors, cases with cystic morphology and predominant mucous cells; however, in some series, no statistical significance was found (Luk et al. 2016; Birkeland et al. 2017) (Fig. 7.1). Lymph node metastasis is rare and may be seen in high-grade tumors.
– *Adenoid cystic carcinoma*:
   The typical morphological pattern of the most frequent submandibular and minor salivary gland malignant tumor is the cribriform pattern (Fig. 7.2). Tubular and solid patterns are the other types. Microscopically invasion beyond the grossly visible margins is frequent. Half of the adenoid cystic carcinomas exhibit a t(6;9) translocation resulting in a MYB-NFIB gene fusion (West et al. 2011). Perineural invasion is frequent in this type of tumor, and it was identified in about half of the cases; but, it was not among the independent prognostics in some series (Jang et al. 2017). However, about a quarter of these cases with neural invasion were found to have intraneural invasion in a series by Amit et al. (2015), and this was identified as a poor prognostic marker for both overall and disease-free survival (hazard ratio of 1.8 and 5.9, respectively), but not for distant metastasis in multivariate analysis. Also perineural invasion of the large nerves was identified as a poor prognostic factor (Fig. 7.3).

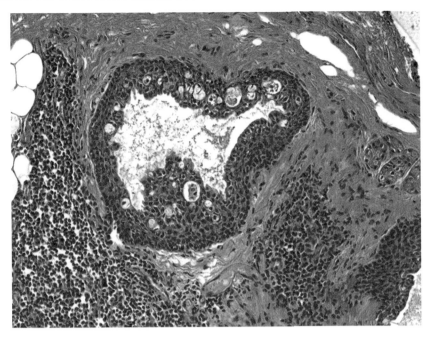

Fig. 7.1 Mucinous, intermediate and epidermoid cells arranged in cystic and solid areas make up the tumor mass (H&E, original magnification ×20)

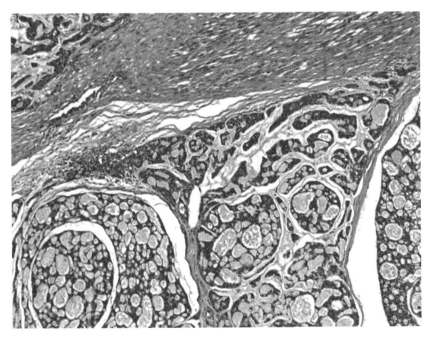

Fig. 7.2 Cribriform pattern of adenoid cystic carcinoma, which is the most frequent (H&E, original magnification ×20)

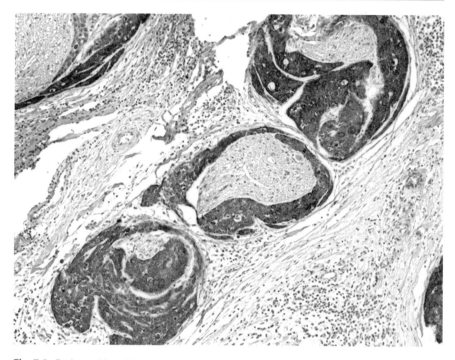

Fig. 7.3 Perineural invasion, solid-type adenoid cystic carcinoma, and intraneural and perineural invasion at the lower part (IHC, keratin, original magnification ×20)

– *Acinic cell carcinoma*:

The parotid gland is the most frequent site for acinic cell carcinoma, and finely granular, basophilic cytoplasm resembling the normal acinar cells is the characteristic feature. Mixed cellular and morphological pattern is the characteristic feature of these tumors. Serous, oncocytic, basaloid, clear-cells and acinar, microcystic, follicular, papillary, and solid growth patterns may be seen (Fig. 7.4). Strong, granular cytoplasmic PAS positivity in the acinar type and amylase, antichymotrypsin, and DOG-1 expressions may help diagnosis. Mammary analogue secretory carcinoma should be in the differential diagnosis (Said-Al-Naief et al. 2017). In cases with dedifferentiation, poor outcome is expected; otherwise lymph node metastasis and distant metastasis is seen in less than 10% of the cases.

– *Polymorphous adenocarcinoma*:

Lobular growth pattern, cytological uniformity, and morphological diversity are the characteristic features of this tumor. p40 negative staining and positivity of myoepithelial markers, such as mammaglobin, CEA, GFAP, galectin 3, and bcl2, may help differential diagnosis (Rooper et al. 2015; Argyris et al. 2016). *HRAS* mutations and *PRKD* gene family rearrangements were found in polymorphous carcinoma cases. In the WHO 2017 classification of head and neck tumors, instead of "polymorphous low-grade adenocarcinoma" terminology, "polymorphous adenocarcinoma" was used, considering the cases which may not be low grade. These tumors may not be low grade, or they may have high-grade transformation (Seethala and Stenman 2017).

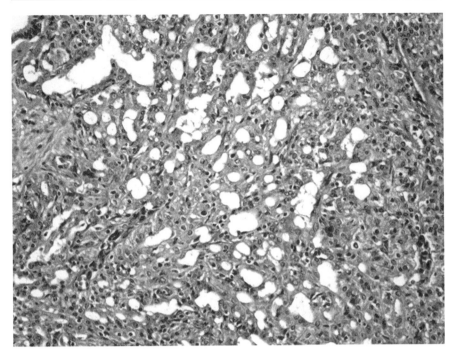

Fig. 7.4 Acinic cell carcinoma with typical morphological features forming acinar and microfollicular patterns (H&E, original magnification ×20)

- *Clear-cell carcinoma:*
  A tumor made of p63-positive clear cells and negative myoepithelial markers; hyalinized stroma is a characteristic feature of this tumor. It is most frequently seen in intraoral salivary glands. *EWSR1-ATF1* fusion is consistent (Antonescu et al. 2011).
- *Basal cell adenocarcinoma:*
  This rare tumor mimics basal cell adenoma with basement membrane-like material, palisading basaloid and myoepithelial cells. Mitosis, invasion, and metastasis are features of malignancy.
- *Salivary duct carcinoma:*
  Salivary duct carcinoma resembling high-grade mammary ductal carcinoma is an aggressive tumor with large, atypical cells forming Roman bridges, cribriform pattern, and comedo necrosis. Sarcomatoid, mucin-rich, micropapillary, and oncocytic variants may be seen. Androgen receptor positivity is seen in 70–86%, and HER2 positivity is seen in 25–30% of the cases. Because of these features, targeted therapy possibilities are being evaluated (Dalin et al. 2017; Thorpe et al. 2017). Intraductal carcinoma should be in the differential diagnosis which have significantly better prognosis (Fig. 7.5).
- *Myoepithelial carcinoma:*
  This rare tumor may be composed of plasmacytoid, epithelioid, spindle, and clear cells forming solid, trabecular, and reticular patterns. *EWSR1* gene rearrangement is seen in this case (Skalova et al. 2015).

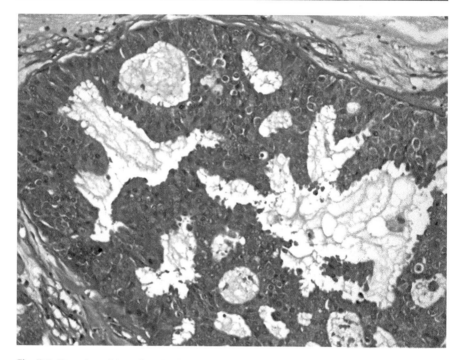

Fig. 7.5 Ductal carcinoma forming Roman bridges and cribriform pattern. Invasion is in favor of ductal carcinoma (H&E, original magnification ×40)

- *Epithelial-myoepithelial carcinoma:*
  Lacelike pattern composed of glandular structures delineated by epithelial cells at the luminal and clear myoepithelial cells at the abluminal parts (Fig. 7.6). This carcinoma with favorable prognosis has no genetic landmarks (Vázquez et al. 2015).
- *Carcinoma ex pleomorphic adenoma:*
  Most of the malignant tumors arising from pleomorphic adenomas are not otherwise specified adenocarcinomas, ductal carcinomas, and myoepithelial carcinomas. In addition to *PLAG1* and *HMGA2* fusion genes in pleomorphic adenomas, *TP53* mutation and *MDM2, HMGA2,* and *HER2* amplifications are frequent in cases with malignant transformation (Thorpe et al. 2017) (Fig. 7.7).
- *Secretory carcinoma*:
  This tumor is included in the last WHO classification. Previously, this tumor was misdiagnosed as acinic cell carcinoma. Microcystic/solid, tubular, follicular, and papillary cystic structures with luminal secretion are the typical features of the tumor. t(12;15)(p13;q25) translocation resulting in *ETV6-NTRK3* fusion seen in breast secretory carcinomas is the hallmark of this tumor (Skálová et al. 2010). S100 and mammaglobin positivity and DOG-1 negativity may help differential diagnosis.

Sebaceous, neuroendocrine carcinomas, squamous cell carcinoma, oncocytic carcinoma, sialoblastoma, and carcinosarcoma are rare but should be kept in mind. Lymphoepithelial carcinoma is rare but has a geographic distribution, and Epstein-Barr virus plays an important role in pathogenesis and helps diagnosis (Figs. 7.8 and 7.9).

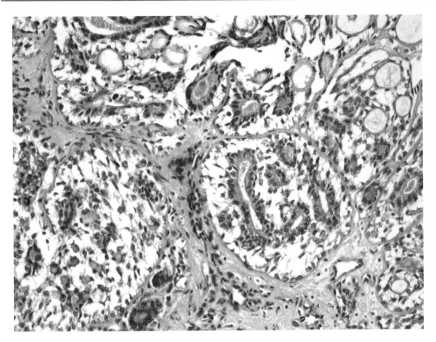

Fig. 7.6 Typical morphology of epithelial-myoepithelial carcinoma (H&E, original magnification ×20)

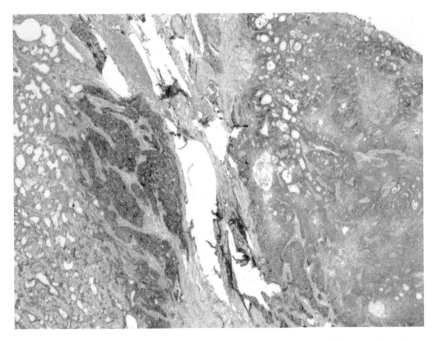

Fig. 7.7 Carcinoma ex pleomorphic adenoma. At the left side, at the site of pleomorphic adenoma, cerbB2 expression is negative or minimally positive, but at the right side, at the site of ductal carcinoma, ++/+++ cytoplasmic membranous positive staining is seen (H&E, original magnification ×10)

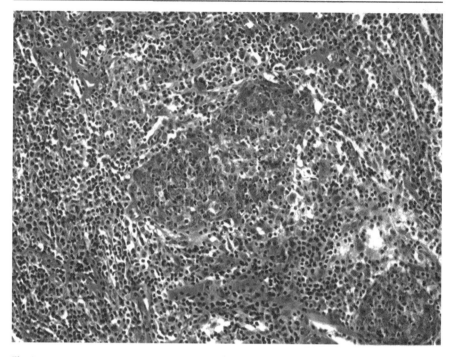

Fig. 7.8 Lymphoepithelial carcinoma: infiltration of the neoplastic cells with many lymphocytes (H&E, original magnification ×20)

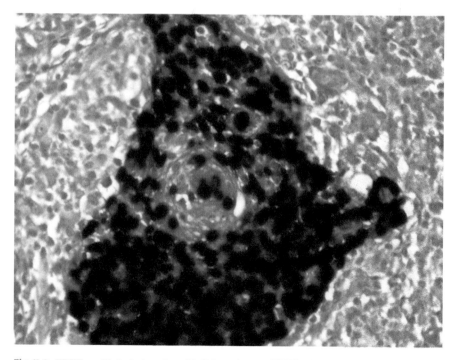

Fig. 7.9 EBER positivity in lymphoepithelial carcinoma (CISH, original magnification ×40)

Prognostic Factors in Salivary Gland Carcinomas

The prognosis of salivary gland tumors was evaluated either as case series including all types of salivary gland tumors or series of a single type of carcinoma. Many prognostic factors including histopathological features were evaluated in a series of 565 malignant parotid gland tumors by Terhaard et al. (2004). In this large series, in multivariate analysis, independent factors for distant metastasis were sex, T and N stage, perineural invasion, and histopathological type. Age, sex, T and pN stage, primary tumor location, and skin and bone invasion were independent prognostic factors for overall survival. Walvekar et al. (2011) identified extracapsular spread of the metastatic lymph nodes and margin status as independent predictors of disease-free survival in 115 cases. In the series of 127 parotid carcinoma cases by Carillo et al., age, facial palsy, tumor type and grade, and surgical margins were the risk factors for recurrences (Carrillo et al. 2007). Mariano et al. (2011) worked on a series of 255 major salivary gland tumors; submandibular gland tumors had twice more common lymph node metastasis compared with the parotid and sublingual glands, and the highest risk for distant metastasis was found for adenoid cystic carcinoma cases.

Histopathological tumor type may have some relation to tumor grade; however, considering unexpected behaviors of some tumors that once were thought of as low grade, careful tumor grading should be exercised (Seethala 2011). Also high-grade transformation in salivary gland tumors is an important issue, and it may be seen in adenoid cystic carcinoma, polymorphous carcinoma, acinic cell carcinoma and mammary analogue secretory carcinoma cases, resulting in poor survival. Molecular markers are important in both diagnosis and prognosis of salivary gland tumors. CRTC1-MALM2 gene fusion in mucoepidermoid carcinoma may be an important prognostic marker of better prognosis; however, there are controversial results in different series (Luk et al. 2016; Birkeland et al. 2017).

Considering many types of salivary gland tumors, the prognostic factors in each type of tumor present some differences, but it is beyond the scope of this chapter.

Discussion About TDs in Salivary Gland Carcinomas

Extranodal tumor metastasis or tumor deposits or soft tissue deposits are lesions which may be a component of tumor progression in many types of carcinoma. They were first recognized in colorectal carcinomas (Nagtegaal et al. 2011; Puppa et al. 2009; Shimada and Takii 2010) than they were observed in many types of carcinomas like gastric carcinomas (Etoh et al. 2006; Ersen et al. 2014; Jiang et al. 2014; Chen et al. 2016) as well as head and neck squamous cell carcinomas (Jose et al. 2004, Kelder et al. 2012; Jose et al. 2007; Sinha et al. 2015, Sarioglu et al. 2016). Do salivary gland carcinomas produce free tumor deposits?

There is only one series answering this question to the best of our knowledge. We have recently evaluated the TDs in a series of 25 salivary gland carcinomas with neck dissection specimens and prognostic information. Seven patients (28%) had TDs. We observed TDs in adenoid cystic carcinoma, basaloid adenocarcinoma, salivary duct carcinoma, and carcinoma ex-pleomorphic adenoma cases. Although there was not a significant difference for the cases with TDs and the others for well known clinicopathological prognostic parameters, disease-free and overall survival of the cases with TD were shorter, without statistical significance. The number of cases in our series was small to draw strict conclusions. The different histopathological types of salivary gland tumors made the issue more complicated. However, this series is valuable for providing the documentation of TDs in salivary gland tumors and the tendency for the poor prognosis of the cases with TDs (Sarioglu S, et al. in press).

A few examples from our cases are presented here: adenoid cystic carcinoma, lymphoepithelioma, and basal cell adenocarcinoma (Figs. 7.10, 7.11, 7.12, and 7.13). Metastatic lymph nodes should always be in the differential diagnosis of these lesions, and metastatic lesions should be evaluated for lymph node structures (Fig. 7.14).

These findings highlight the existence of tumor deposits in salivary gland tumors. Considering they are among the worst prognostic factors in different types of carcinomas, large series of salivary gland malignant tumor cases should be evaluated for tumor deposits and their prognostic implications.

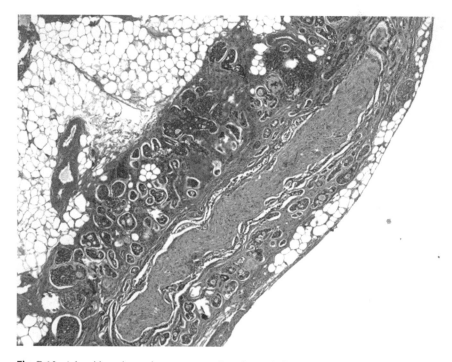

Fig. 7.10 Adenoid cystic carcinoma metastasis at the neck dissection specimen. The deposit is at the perineural region forming a tumor deposit

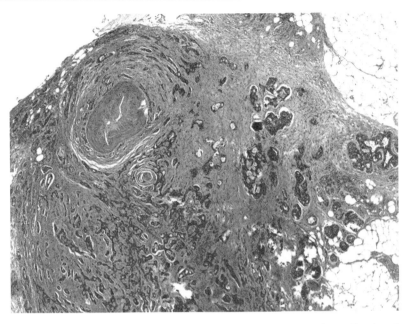

Fig. 7.11 Adenoid cystic carcinoma metastasis in the neck dissection specimen. The deposit was probably formed by extravascular perivascular migratory pathway (H&E, original magnification ×20)

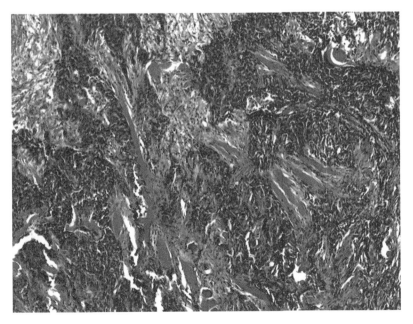

Fig. 7.12 Free tumor deposit from the lymphoepithelioma. The free tumor deposit was metastatic from the parotid gland tumor and was invading the striated muscles of the neck. Epstein-Barr virus-encoded RNA chromogenic in situ hybridization was positive in the neck dissection specimen (H&E, original magnification ×20)

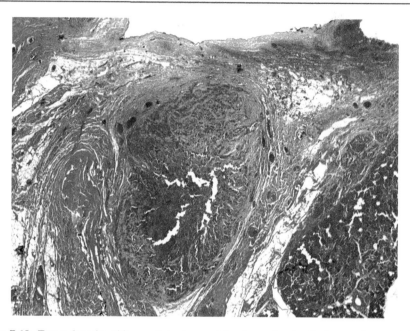

Fig. 7.13 Tumor deposits with smooth contours arising from a basal cell adenocarcinoma of the parotid gland. The basement membrane material and palisading of the epithelial cells can be seen at the tumor deposit. It is hard to speculate about the mechanism of the formation of this deposit; there are no lymph node structures, peripheral nerves, or blood vessels. However serial sections may provide further evidence (H&E, original magnification ×20)

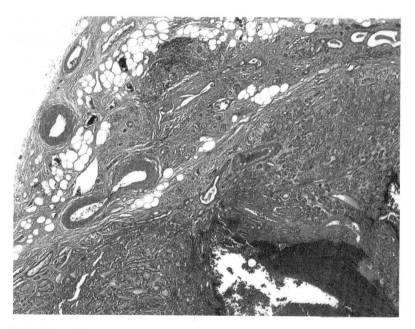

Fig. 7.14 Metastatic basal cell adenocarcinoma with perinodal invasion. This image may resemble a free tumor deposit with regular contours of the perivascular type; however, it was from a metastatic lymph node replaced by metastatic adenocarcinoma, but about two-thirds of the lymph node structure was retained

References

Amit M, Binenbaum Y, Trejo-Leider L, Sharma K, Ramer N, Ramer I, Agbetoba A, Miles B, Yang X, Lei D, Bjørndal K, Godballe C, Mücke T, Wolff KD, Eckardt AM, Copelli C, Sesenna E, Palmer F, Ganly I, Patel S, Gil Z. International collaborative validation of intraneural invasion as a prognostic marker in adenoid cystic carcinoma of the head and neck. Head Neck. 2015;37(7):1038–45. https://doi.org/10.1002/hed.23710; Epub 2014 Jul 24.

Antonescu CR, Katabi N, Zhang L, Sung YS, Seethala RR, Jordan RC, Perez-Ordoñez B, Have C, Asa SL, Leong IT, Bradley G, Klieb H, Weinreb I. EWSR1-ATF1 fusion is a novel and consistent finding in hyalinizing clear-cell carcinoma of salivary gland. Genes Chromosomes Cancer. 2011;50(7):559–70. https://doi.org/10.1002/gcc.20881; Epub 2011 Apr 11.

Argyris PP, Wetzel SL, Greipp P, Wehrs RN, Knutson DL, Kloft-Nelson SM, García JJ, Koutlas IG. Clinical utility of myb rearrangement detection and p63/p40 immunophenotyping in the diagnosis of adenoid cystic carcinoma of minor salivary glands: a pilot study. Oral Surg Oral Med Oral Pathol Oral Radiol. 2016;121(3):282–9. https://doi.org/10.1016/j.oooo.2015.10.016; Epub 2015 Oct 19.

Birkeland AC, Foltin SK, Michmerhuizen NL, Hoesli RC, Rosko AJ, Byrd S, Yanik M, Nor JE, Bradford CR, Prince ME, Carey TE, McHugh JB, Spector ME, Brenner JC. Correlation of Crtc1/3-Maml2 fusion status, grade and survival in mucoepidermoid carcinoma. Oral Oncol. 2017;68:5–8. https://doi.org/10.1016/j.oraloncology.2017.02.025; Epub 2017 Mar 10.

Carrillo JF, Vázquez R, Ramírez-Ortega MC, Cano A, Ochoa-Carrillo FJ, Oñate-Ocaña LF. Multivariate prediction of the probability of recurrence in patients with carcinoma of the parotid gland. Cancer. 2007;109(10):2043–51.

Chen XL, Zhao LY, Xue L, Xu YH, Zhang WH, Liu K, Chen XZ, Yang K, Zhang B, Chen ZX, Chen JP, Zhou ZG, Hu JK. Prognostic significance and the role in TNM stage of extranodal metastasis within regional lymph nodes station in gastric carcinoma. Oncotarget. 2016;7(41):67047–60. 10.18632/oncotarget.11478.

Dalin MG, Watson PA, Ho AL, Morris LG. Androgen receptor signaling in salivary gland cancer. Cancers (Basel). 2017;9(2). https://doi.org/10.3390/cancers9020017. Review.

Etit D, Tan A, Bakir K, Cakalagaoglu F, Elagoz S, Elpek GO, Han O, Han U, Hucumenoglu S, Koybasioglu F, Kucuk U, Kulacoglu S, Paker I, Sarioglu S, Seckin S, Tekkesin MS, Uguz A, Unal T, Gunhan O. Interobserver agreement in salivary gland neoplasms by telepathology: an analysis of 47 cases. Anal Quant Cytopathol Histpathol. 2013;35(2):114–20.

Ersen A, Unlu MS, Akman T, Sagol O, Oztop I, Atila K, Bora S, Ellidokuz H, Sarioglu S. Tumor deposits in gastric carcinomas. Pathol Res Pract. 2014;210(9):565–70. https://doi.org/10.1016/j.prp.2014.03.006; Epub 2014 Mar 27.

Etoh T, Sasako M, Ishikawa K, Katai H, Sano T, Shimoda T. Extranodal metastasis is an indicator of poor prognosis in patients with gastric carcinoma. Br J Surg. 2006;93(3):369–73.

Foschini MP, Morandi L, Asioli S, Giove G, Corradini AG, Eusebi V. The morphological spectrum of salivary gland type tumours of the breast. Pathology. 2017;49(2):215–27. https://doi.org/10.1016/j.pathol.2016.10.011; Epub 2016 Dec 30. Review.

Gibault L, Badoual C. [Salivary gland-type lung tumor: an update]. Ann Pathol 2016;36(1):55–62. doi: https://doi.org/10.1016/j.annpat.2015.11.003; Epub 2016 Jan 7. Review. French.

Jang S, Patel PN, Kimple RJ, McCulloch TM. Clinical outcomes and prognostic factors of adenoid cystic carcinoma of the head and neck. Anticancer Res. 2017;37(6):3045–52.

Jiang N, Deng JY, Ding XW, Ke B, Liu N, Liang H. Node-extranodal soft tissue stage based on extranodal metastasis is associated with poor prognosis of patients with gastric cancer. J Surg Res. 2014;192(1):90–7. https://doi.org/10.1016/j.jss.2014.05.053; Epub 2014 May 23.

Jose J, Moor JW, Coatesworth AP, Johnston C, MacLennan K. Soft tissue deposits in neck dissections of patients with head and neck squamous cell carcinoma: prospective analysis of prevalence, survival, and its implications. Arch Otolaryngol Head Neck Surg. 2004;130(2):157–60.

Jose J, Ferlito A, Rodrigo JP, Devaney KO, Rinaldo A, MacLennan K. Soft tissue deposits from head and neck cancer: an under-recognised prognostic factor? J Laryngol Otol. 2007;121(12):1115–7.

Kalhor N, Weissferdt A, Moran CA. Primary Salivary Gland Type Tumors of the Thymus. Adv Anat Pathol. 2017;24(1):15–23. Review.

Kelder W, Ebrahimi A, Forest VI, Gao K, Murali R, Clark JR. Cutaneous head and neck squamous cell carcinoma with regional metastases: the prognostic importance of soft tissue metastases and extranodal spread. Ann Surg Oncol. 2012;19(1):274–9. https://doi.org/10.1245/s10434-011-1986-7; Epub 2011 Aug 9.

Mariano FV, da Silva SD, Chulan TC, de Almeida OP, Kowalski LP. Clinicopathological factors are predictors of distant metastasis from major salivary gland carcinomas. Int J Oral Maxillofac Surg. 2011;40(5):504–9. https://doi.org/10.1016/j.ijom.2010.12.002.

Luk PP, Wykes J, Selinger CI, Ekmejian R, Tay J, Gao K, Eviston TJ, Lum T, O'Toole SA, Clark JR, Gupta R. Diagnostic and prognostic utility of Mastermind-like 2 (MAML2) gene rearrangement detection by fluorescent in situ hybridization (FISH) in mucoepidermoid carcinoma of the salivary glands. Oral Surg Oral Med Oral Pathol Oral Radiol. 2016;121(5):530–41. https://doi.org/10.1016/j.oooo.2016.01.003; Epub 2016 Jan 9.

Nagtegaal ID, Tot T, Jayne DG, McShane P, Nihlberg A, Marshall HC, Påhlman L, Brown JM, Guillou PJ, Quirke P. Lymph nodes, tumor deposits, and TNM: are we getting better? J Clin Oncol. 2011;29(18):2487–92. https://doi.org/10.1200/JCO.2011.34.6429; Epub 2011 May 9.

Puppa G, Ueno H, Kayahara M, Capelli P, Canzonieri V, Colombari R, Maisonneuve P, Pelosi G. Tumor deposits are encountered in advanced colorectal cancer and other adenocarcinomas: an expanded classification with implications for colorectal cancer staging system including a unifying concept of in-transit metastases. Mod Pathol. 2009;22(3):410–5. https://doi.org/10.1038/modpathol.2008.198; Epub 2009 Jan 9.

Rooper L, Sharma R, Bishop JA. Polymorphous low grade adenocarcinoma has a consistent p63+/p40- immunophenotype that helps distinguish it from adenoid cystic carcinoma and cellular pleomorphic adenoma. Head Neck Pathol. 2015;9(1):79–84. https://doi.org/10.1007/s12105-014-0554-4; Epub 2014 Jun 27.

Said-Al-Naief N, Carlos R, Vance GH, Miller C, Edwards PC. Combined DOG1 and mammaglobin immunohistochemistry is comparable to ETV6-breakapart analysis for differentiating between papillary cystic variants of acinic cell carcinoma and mammary analogue secretory carcinoma. Int J Surg Pathol. 2017;25(2):127–40. https://doi.org/10.1177/1066896916670005; Epub 2016 Sep 26.

Sarioglu S, Kilicarslan E, Aydin B, Kozen MA, Akman F, Oztop I, Ada E, İkiz AO. Tumor deposits in salivary gland tumors. Pathol Int. (in press).

Sarioglu S, Akbulut N, Iplikci S, Aydin B, Dogan E, Unlu M, Ellidokuz H, Ada E, Akman F, Ikiz AO. Tumor deposits in head and neck carcinomas. Head Neck. 2016;38(Suppl 1):E256–60. https://doi.org/10.1002/hed.23981; Epub 2015 Aug 21.

Seethala RR. Histologic grading and prognostic biomarkers in salivary gland carcinomas. Adv Anat Pathol. 2011;18(1):29–45. https://doi.org/10.1097/PAP.0b013e318202645a. Review.

Seethala RR, Stenman G. Update from the 4th Edition of the World Health Organization Classification of head and neck tumours: tumors of the salivary gland. Head Neck Pathol. 2017;11(1):55–67. https://doi.org/10.1007/s12105-017-0795-0; Epub 2017 Feb 28.

Shimada Y, Takii Y. Clinical impact of mesorectal extranodal cancer tissue in rectal cancer: detailed pathological assessment using whole-mount sections. Dis Colon Rectum. 2010;53(5):771–8. https://doi.org/10.1007/DCR.0b013e3181cf7fd8.

Sinha P, Lewis JS Jr, Kallogjeri D, Nussenbaum B, Haughey BH. Soft tissue metastasis in p16-positive oropharynx carcinoma: prevalence and association with distant metastasis. Oral Oncol. 2015;51(8):778–86. https://doi.org/10.1016/j.oraloncology.2015.05.004; Epub 2015 May 29.

Skálová A, Vanecek T, Sima R, Laco J, Weinreb I, Perez-Ordonez B, Starek I, Geierova M, Simpson RH, Passador-Santos F, Ryska A, Leivo I, Kinkor Z, Michal M. Mammary analogue secretory carcinoma of salivary glands, containing the ETV6-NTRK3 fusion gene: a hitherto undescribed salivary gland tumor entity. Am J Surg Pathol. 2010;34(5):599–608. https://doi.org/10.1097/PAS.0b013e3181d9efcc.

Skálová A, Weinreb I, Hyrcza M, Simpson RH, Laco J, Agaimy A, Vazmitel M, Majewska H, Vanecek T, Talarčik P, Manajlovic S, Losito SN, Šteiner P, Klimkova A, Michal M. Clear cell myoepithelial carcinoma of salivary glands showing EWSR1 rearrangement: molecular analysis of 94 salivary gland carcinomas with prominent clear cell component. Am J Surg Pathol. 2015;39(3):338–48. https://doi.org/10.1097/PAS.0000000000000364.

Sobin LH, Gospodarowicz MK, Wittekind CH, editors. International Union against cancer. TNM classification of malignant tumours. 7th ed. West Sussex, England: Wiley-Blackwell; 2009.

Terhaard CH, Lubsen H, Van der Tweel I, Hilgers FJ, Eijkenboom WM, Marres HA, Tjho-Heslinga RE, de Jong JM, Roodenburg JL, Dutch Head and Neck Oncology Cooperative Group. Salivary gland carcinoma: independent prognostic factors for locoregional control, distant metastases, and overall survival: results of the Dutch head and neck oncology cooperative group. Head Neck. 2004;26(8):681–92; discussion 692–3.

Thorpe LM, Schrock AB, Erlich RL, Miller VA, Knost J, Le-Lindqwister N, Jujjavarapu S, Ali SM, Liu JJ. Significant and durable clinical benefit from trastuzumab in 2 patients with HER2-amplified salivary gland cancer and a review of the literature. Head Neck. 2017;39(3):E40–4. https://doi.org/10.1002/hed.24634; Epub 2016 Dec 22.

Vázquez A, Patel TD, D'Aguillo CM, Abdou RY, Farver W, Baredes S, Eloy JA, Park RC. Epithelial-myoepithelial carcinoma of the salivary glands: an analysis of 246 cases. Otolaryngol Head Neck Surg. 2015;153(4):569–74. https://doi.org/10.1177/0194599815594788; Epub 2015 Jul 20.

Walvekar RR, Andrade Filho PA, Seethala RR, Gooding WE, Heron DE, Johnson JT, Ferris RL. Clinicopathologic features as stronger prognostic factors than histology or grade in risk stratification of primary parotid malignancies. Head Neck. 2011;33(2):225–31.

West RB, Kong C, Clarke N, Gilks T, Lipsick JS, Cao H, Kwok S, Montgomery KD, Varma S, Le QT. MYB expression and translocation in adenoid cystic carcinomas and other salivary gland tumors with clinicopathologic correlation. Am J Surg Pathol. 2011;35(1):92–9. https://doi.org/10.1097/PAS.0b013e3182002777.

Tumor Deposits in Head and Neck Tumors

8

The most frequent type of head and neck tumors is squamous cell carcinomas (SCC), and the variants of SCC are not frequent. The prognosis of carcinomas with similar histology at different sites of the head and neck is different.

The search for prognostic factors of the head and neck carcinomas is still in progress. The last classification of the tumors of the head and neck has been expanded including new entities. Nasal cavity and paranasal sinus, larynx and pharynx, oral cavity, and oropharynx carcinomas are classified histopathologically as separate entities, and there are differences between the tumor types according to the primary sites.

There are a few studies about the tumor deposits in head and neck carcinomas with prognostic information. In this chapter, types of head and neck tumors are briefly presented along with prognostic information as well as the information about the tumor deposits as prognostic factors.

Morphologic and Molecular Classifications of the Head and Neck Carcinomas

Nasal Cavity and the Paranasal Sinuses

Non-keratinizing squamous cell carcinomas (NKSCC) of the nasal cavity are more frequent than the keratinizing type (KSCC), and chemical carcinogens like cigarette smoking are more frequent in the former one, while 50% of NKSCC are positive for high-risk human papillomavirus (Figs. 8.1 and 8.2).

There are rare variants of sinonasal carcinomas which are both HPV and EBV negative, like intestinal-type and non-intestinal-type adenocarcinomas, spindle cell carcinomas, SMARCB-1 (INI-1)-deficient carcinomas, nuclear protein in testis (NUT) gene (*NUTM1*) rearrangement carcinomas, and sinonasal undifferentiated carcinomas (Fig. 8.3). On the other hand, sinonasal tract HPV-related carcinomas with adenoid cystic-like features and lymphoepithelial carcinomas which are EBV positive in 90% of the cases are related to viral infections (Figs. 8.4 and 8.5). Neuroendocrine carcinomas are rare and rarely related to HPV (Slootweg and Grandis 2017).

© Springer International Publishing AG 2018
S. Sarioglu, *Tumor Deposits*, https://doi.org/10.1007/978-3-319-68582-3_8

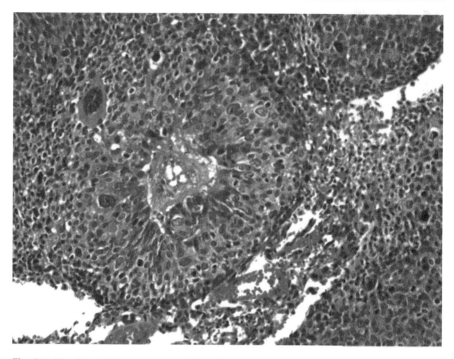

Fig. 8.1 Non-keratinizing squamous cell carcinoma mimicking inverted papilloma, but there is severe atypia and invasion (H&E, original magnification ×40)

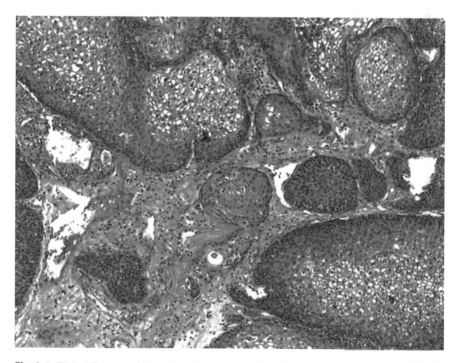

Fig. 8.2 Well-differentiated keratinizing squamous cell carcinoma of the frontal sinus with brain invasion (H&E, original magnification ×40)

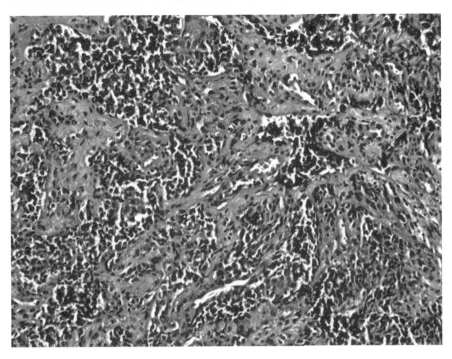

Fig. 8.3 Sinonasal undifferentiated carcinoma, a diagnosis requiring exclusion of many types of carcinomas (H&E, original magnification ×20)

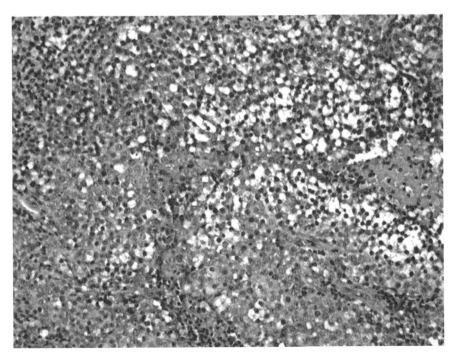

Fig. 8.4 Lymphoepithelial carcinoma with many infiltrating lymphocytes (H&E, original magnification ×20)

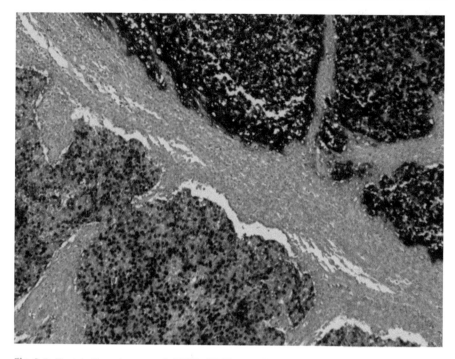

Fig. 8.5 Epstein-Barr virus-encoded RNA (EBER) positivity in sinonasal lymphoepithelial carcinoma (EBER chromagen in situ hybridization, original magnification ×20)

Oral Cavity, Larynx, Hypopharynx, and Trachea

The most frequent type of carcinoma of these regions is conventional SCC. SCC variants and rare epithelial tumors include verrucous, basaloid, papillary, spindle cell, adenosquamous, and lymphoepithelial carcinomas (Figs. 8.6, 8.7, 8.8, and 8.9). Cigarette smoking and chewing tobacco and betel quid are the most frequent etiological factors, and loss of tumor suppressor genes like *CDKN2A* and *TP53* is frequent as well as mutation in the oncogenes. HPV infection may be an etiological factor at these sites, most common at the conventional type, but less frequent than the oropharyngeal region.

Oropharynx

At the last edition of the WHO classification, the oropharyngeal SCC are classified as HPV positive and negative (El-Naggar and Takata 2017). HPV-positive cases are distinctly different from the others. Small primary non-keratinizing SCC arising from the deep cryptic regions giving rise to cystic lymph node metastasis of the neck in male patients at the median age 50–56 are a typical feature of these cases. p16 protein expression related to E7 inactivation of the RB and somatic mutation of the *TRAF3* are unique for HPV(+) oral SCC, and amplification of the oncogene *PIK3CA* is frequent in these cases (Figs. 8.10, 8.11, and 8.12) (El-Naggar AK and Takata 2017).

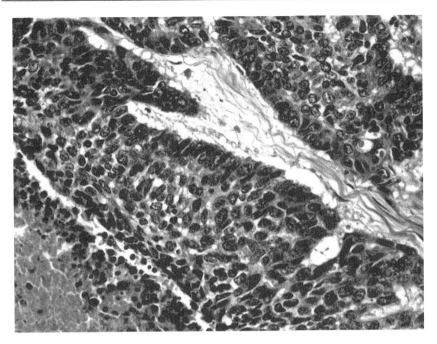

Fig. 8.6 Basaloid SCC of the larynx with basaloid cells and peripheral palisading (H&E, original magnification ×40)

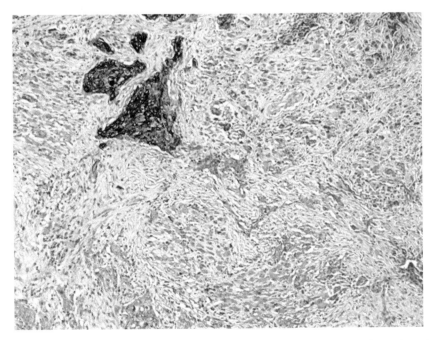

Fig. 8.7 Spindle cell carcinoma with loss of keratin expression in many cells which are vimentin positive (Pan-keratin, original magnification ×20) (Fig. 8.8)

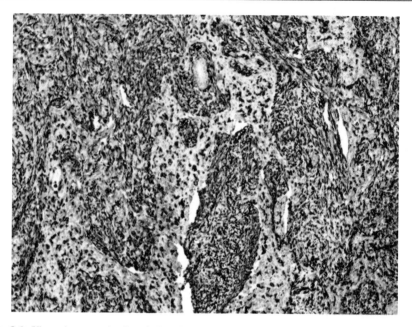

Fig. 8.8 Vimentin expression in spindle cell carcinoma (Vimentin, original magnification ×20)

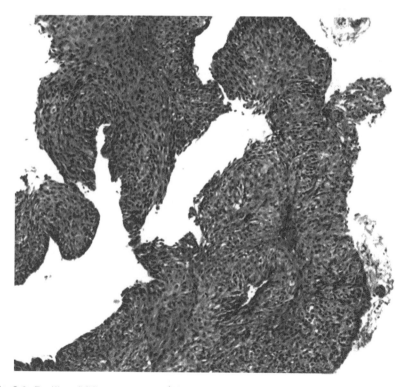

Fig. 8.9 Papillary SCC, a rare variant (H&E, original magnification ×10)

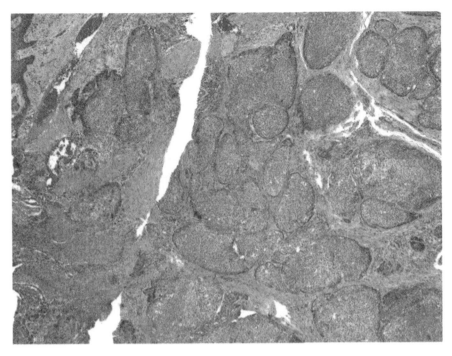

Fig. 8.10 Non-keratinizing squamous cell carcinoma of the oropharynx (H&E, original magnification ×10)

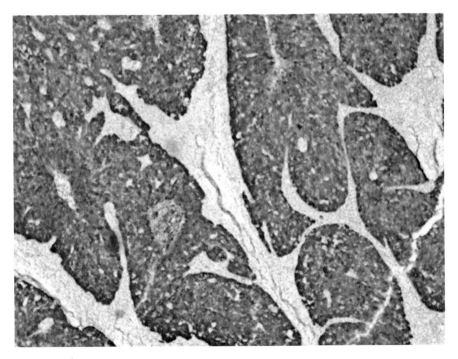

Fig. 8.11 Strong p16 protein expression in non-keratinizing squamous cell carcinoma of the oropharynx (IHC, p16, original magnification ×20)

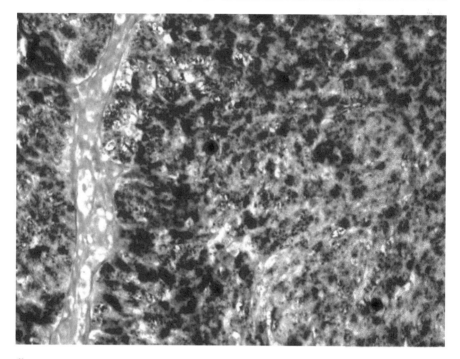

Fig. 8.12 Non-keratinizing squamous cell carcinoma of the oropharynx (chromagen in situ hybridization, high-risk HPV, original magnification ×40)

Prognostic Factors in Head and Neck Carcinomas

Many histopathological prognostic factors have been described for head and neck carcinomas. Tumors arising from the different parts of the larynx and oral cavity have different prognostic features as well as those from the nasal cavity and the paranasal sinuses. In standard pathology reports, tumor location; histopathological type; pathological T stage; distance from the tumor to the closest surgical margin; perineural, vascular, and lymphatic invasion; and tumor budding should be noted. Lymph node metastasis and perinodal invasion are also important prognostic features of head and neck carcinomas like many types of carcinomas.

We have identified T and N stage, EGFR expression, and tumor budding in different laryngeal carcinoma series, but tumor-stroma ratio was not identified as a poor prognostic factor (Demiral et al. 2004; Nur et al. 2005; Sarioglu et al. 2010; Unlu et al. 2013). Treatment center may also be a prognostic factor for the head and neck carcinomas (Akman et al. 2008). Early and late SCC of the laryngeal carcinomas have different features and different treatment modalities.

Proposed Mechanisms and Morphology of Tumor Deposits in Head and Neck Carcinomas

In the series by Violaris et al. (1994), the free soft tissue masses in neck dissection specimens were more frequently found in patients with poor general condition, poorly differentiated carcinomas, and carcinomas at T4 stage, and they suggested that these features played a role in the development, but they did not suggest any mechanism at the cellular level.

Jose et al. (2003) suggested that the soft tissue deposits might represent extralymphatic deposits of SCC or a totally effaced lymph node. In 2004, Jose et al., along with a series of head and neck carcinoma cases with prognostic information, made further comments about the soft tissue deposits in head and neck SCC cases. They suggested that SCC spread from the primary tumor may be by embolization, lymphatic invasion, or neural route and the metastatic tumor cells at the lymph nodes which proliferate and replace the whole lymph node structure or extravasate out of the lymphatic channels to form deposits, reflecting the more aggressive properties of the cells forming tumor deposits.

Cabanillas et al. (2005) presented an animal model of SCC in nude mice and identified tumor deposits in neck specimens. All 20 mice injected with human laryngeal SCC cells developed tumors with perineural invasion and lymph node metastasis, and the authors reported that they identified tumor cells escaping the lymphatics or traveling through small vessels and ending up as free tumor deposits in the soft tissues.

Kelder et al. (2012) suggested that the tumor deposits in head and neck SCC were not lymph nodes completely replaced by tumor, but they represented a distinct biologic entity. They compared the TDs with satellitosis in malignant melanoma cases, and they suggested that these were two separate entities as tumor deposits mainly occurred at the node basins rather than as dermal deposits close to the primary tumor. However, they highlighted the requirement of a strict definition for tumor deposits like the satellitosis lesions of the melanoma cases. They also agreed with the previous reports about the alternative pathways for tumor deposit formation, through lymphatic channels and perineural or vascular routes. They suggested that malignant cells escaping lymphatic channels might possess properties of increased growth and dissemination and escape the immune regulatory mechanisms that are part of the lymph node functions. However, they noted that the real explanation might be complicated and multifactorial.

Sinha et al. (2015) evaluated the prognostic value of soft tissue metastasis from oropharyngeal carcinomas in a series of 222 p16-positive cases. They accepted tumor deposits as the end stage of extranodal spread. They graded extracapsular spread into four grades:

Grade 1 = tumor with smooth leading edge and no extension beyond the capsule

Grade 2 = tumor extending <1 mm beyond the capsule

Grade 3 = tumor extending >1 mm beyond the capsule

Grade 4/soft tissue metastasis (STM) = irregular masses of tumor in the neck soft tissue with no histological evidence of residual lymph node tissue or architecture

In this series, although the authors accepted soft tissue tumors as late stage of extranodal spread, they still noted that some small deposits might be formed by tumor emboli rupturing the lymphatics and extending into the surrounding soft tissue.

In none of the series evaluating the tumor deposits in head and neck carcinomas, a specific mechanism other than the ones proposed for other sites is presented. In our series, we noted that the pathway of the tumor cells may be by intralymphatic or perilymphatic, perivascular, and/or perineural pathways, and, in most cases, this is the result of more than one pathway. We proposed the terminology of "allocated highway," used by tumor cells in order to escape immune system surveillance both at the vessels and the lymph nodes (Sarioglu et al. 2016).

Classifications of Tumor Deposits in Head and Neck Carcinomas

The recognition of soft tissue tumor mass in neck dissection specimens is not very recent, but the issues about classification and definition of risk categories are still a problem. The poor prognostic prediction of tumor deposits arising from oral cavity SCC in neck specimens was reported by Shah in 1976, but they did not present the definition they used for such lesions.

At the study by Violaris et al. (1994), the metastatic lesions in neck dissection specimens were classified as a "free" soft tissue deposit if it was discontinuous with the primary carcinoma and if there was no organized lymphoid tissue at its periphery. They noted that, in most cases, there was desmoplastic response at the periphery of the lesion.

In two studies by Jose et al. (2003) and Jose et al. (2004), lymph node levels were separated from neck dissection specimens, and each was cut into 2 mm thick blocks and sectioned at 6 μm thickness. Lymph nodes were defined as an aggregate of encapsulated lymphoid tissue of any size, which had a peripheral sinus. A soft tissue deposit was defined as SCC in the soft tissues of the neck, without any evidence of a lymph node.

In the series by Kelder et al. (2012) evaluating the tumor deposits arising from cutaneous SCC of the head and neck, STMs were defined as follows: tumor of the soft tissue without continuity with the primary tumor and lacking discernible associated lymph node tissue. The authors excluded metastatic nodes larger than 3 cm and explained this with overcoming the effect of bulky tumors. To exclude the effect of bulky tumors, only patients with metastatic nodes smaller than 3 cm in size were included.

In the series of Sinha et al. (2015), tumor deposits were described as "irregular masses of tumor in the neck soft tissue with no histologic evidence of residual lymph node tissue or architecture." They noted the lack of uniform criteria in the literature about soft tissue metastasis or tumor deposits.

We have also evaluated the prognostic significance of tumor deposits in 140 SCC cases of the head and neck. Any tumor mass either circumscribed or with irregular contours, devoid of lymph node architecture at the neck dissection specimen, was identified as a tumor deposit according to the criteria applied for the colorectal carcinoma cases by the College of American Pathologists Cancer Protocols (CAP 2014). The number of tumor deposits ranged from 1 to 14 and measured 3 to 24 mm.

In none of these series, the metastatic soft tumor deposits or soft tissue tumors were further classified as lesions with irregular or smooth contours and of perineural, perilymphatic, and perivascular types as in the series on colorectal carcinoma (Goldstein and Turner 2000; Ueno et al. 2007). This may be due to the number of cases from different head and neck organs in these series, not allowing multivariate analysis if these parameters are also applied. Some free tumor deposits are presented at Figs. 8.13, 8.14, 8.15, 8.16, 8.17, 8.18, and 8.19.

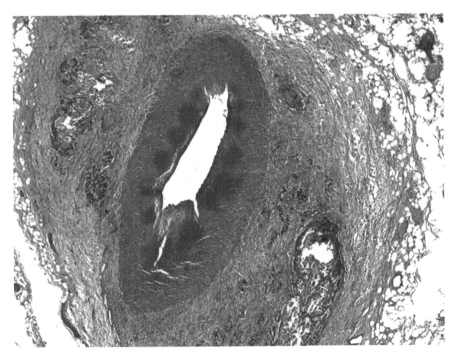

Fig. 8.13 Metastatic squamous cell carcinoma of the larynx forming perivascular tumor deposit. This type of spread seems to be related to perivascular migratory metastasis (H&E, original magnification ×20)

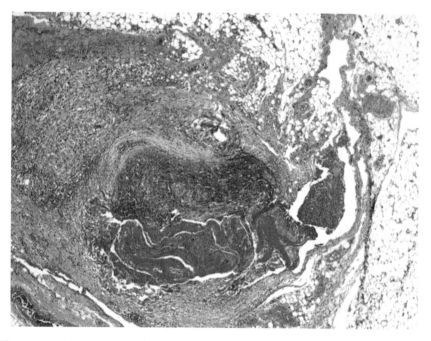

Fig. 8.14 Soft tissue tumor or free tumor deposit at the neck dissection specimen with irregular contours (H&E, original magnification ×20)

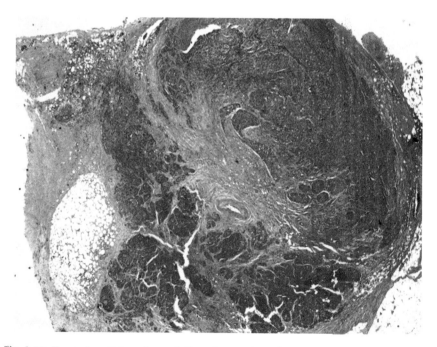

Fig. 8.15 Tumor deposit from the neck dissection specimen from a squamous cell carcinoma of the oral cavity; only vascular structures are identified in this section; this lesion may be related to perivascular invasion (H&E, original magnification ×10)

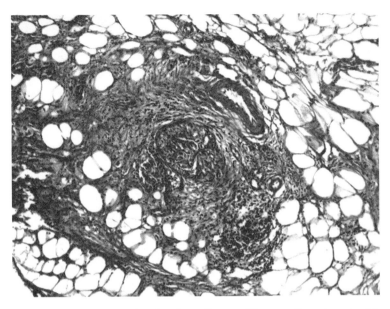

Fig. 8.16 Small soft tissue tumor less than 1 mm diameter. There are discussions about the minimum diameter of lesions that might be diagnosed as tumor deposits; in some series in different organs, it is suggested that lesions smaller than 3 mm should not be classified as tumor deposits (H&E, original magnification ×20)

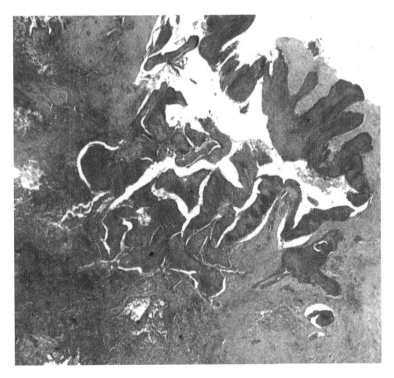

Fig. 8.17 Primary unknown cystic free tumor deposit from the neck of a patient (H&E, original magnification ×4)

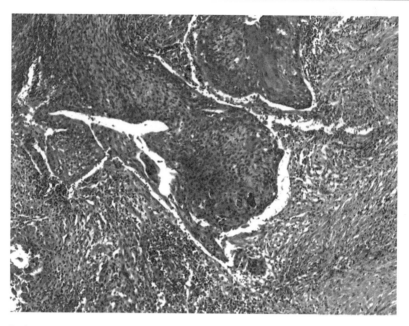

Fig. 8.18 Higher magnification of the case at Fig. 8.17. Note squamous differentiation and peritumoral desmoplastic reaction. No lymph node structure can be identified (H&E, original magnification ×4)

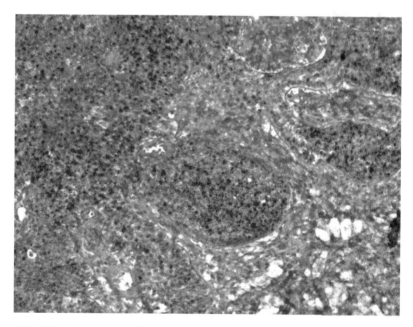

Fig. 8.19 High-risk human papillomavirus in situ hybridization was positive in the case from Figs. 8.17 and 8.18. Although tonsillectomy and base of tongue and nasopharyngeal biopsies were performed prior to the neck mass biopsy, no malignant tumor could be identified (CISH ISH original magnification ×20)

Prognostic Studies on Tumor Deposits in Head and Neck Carcinomas

In the series by Violaris et al. (1994), patients with head and neck carcinomas were evaluated, and the cases were not further classified according to the primary site. Only 497 (16.11%) patients had neck dissection, and in this series, they reported that the patients had either lymph node metastasis or free soft tissue metastasis. They found that 138 (27.77%) cases had soft tissue deposits only and 359 (72.23%) had nodal deposits only. Of the patients with nodal deposits, 165 (45.96%) had perinodal invasion. The 5-year survival rates of the cases with soft tissue metastases, lymph node metastasis with perinodal invasion, and metastatic lymph nodes without perinodal invasion were 27%, 33%, and 50%, respectively. Free soft tissue masses were found more frequently in cases with poorly differentiated SCC cases and T4 tumors. The number of nodes, perinodal invasion, and the presence of free soft tissue metastases were independent prognostic factors in Cox's multivariate analysis.

In the series by Jose et al. (2003), 173 patients with head and neck carcinomas with unilateral or bilateral neck dissection were included, and there were cases from the larynx, hypopharynx, oropharynx, and oral cavity as well as cases with unknown primaries. Perinodal invasion was observed in 37 (21.4%) patients and 42 (23.3%) had soft tissue deposits, while 23 (13.3%) had both extracapsular spread and soft tissue deposits, but there was no prognostic information.

However, in 2004, Jose et al. evaluated the value of soft tissue deposits in a series of 155 patients with head and neck carcinomas. Lymph node metastasis was positive in 65% of the cases, and 23.87% of the cases had tumor deposits. The prognosis of patients with lymph node metastasis and perinodal spread and soft tissue deposits was worse than cases with metastatic lymph nodes. There was no difference between the prognosis of the cases with soft tissue deposits and cases with metastatic lymph nodes with perinodal invasion.

In 2012, in the series by Kelder et al., the tumor deposits arising from cutaneous SCC of the head and neck were identified in 44.5% of the cases in a series of 129 cases with neck dissection. They identified tumor deposits as a significant predictor of reduced overall (hazard ratio = 3.3) and disease-free survival (hazard ratio = 2.4) compared with the patients with lymph node metastasis with or without perinodal invasion.

In a series of 222 p16-positive oropharyngeal SCC cases, Sinha evaluated the prognostic value of soft tissue metastasis. They identified soft tissue metastasis in 55 (27%) cases. Cases with tumor deposits and lymph node metastasis were significantly associated with higher T stage, size of nodal metastasis, and lymphovascular and perineural invasion. Cases with tumor deposits had worse distant metastasis-free survival with a hazard ratio of 4.6 in T3 and T4 cases; however, there was no difference for regional recurrences. For patients who received adjuvant therapy with T3 and T4 tumors with and without tumor deposits, there was no significant difference implying the overcoming potential of poor prognosis by this type of treatment.

In our series of 140 head and neck SCC cases treated with radical surgery and neck dissection, we included cases of larynx, oral cavity, and oropharyngeal carcinoma. Primary tumor of most of the cases was from the larynx [84 cases (60.00%)], followed by the oral cavity [31 cases (22.14%)], hypopharynx [22 cases (15.71%)], and tonsilla palatina [3 cases (0.37%]. Twenty-four patients (17.14%) had tumor deposits. The mean follow-up period in our series was 63.66 ± 54.7 months (range 53–268 months). Locoregional recurrence was seen in 18 patients (12.86%), whereas 6 patients (4.29%) had only local recurrences. There was no difference for tumor deposits when sex, histological type, tumor grade, tumor localization, clinical and pT classifications, surgical margin, perineural invasion, and the number of metastatic lymph nodes were considered. Cases with tumor deposits had more lymphovascular invasion (P=0.007), higher pathological N classification, and distant recurrence. Disease-free survival rates at 12 and 24 months were 93.7% and 85.2%, respectively, for cases without tumor deposits. In cases with tumor deposits, survival rates were 64.1% and 37.9% at 12 and 24 months, respectively. Overall survival rates at 12 and 24 months were 94.2% and 89% for tumor deposit negative cases, and these were 56.8% and 31.6% for tumor deposit positive cases.

Multivariate analysis showed that of all well-known clinicopathological prognostic markers examined, only the presence of tumor deposits showed link to disease-free and overall survival. Cases with tumor deposits had a 2.29-fold increased risk of recurrent disease and were the only independent prognostic indicator to the risk of recurrent disease. Pericapsular invasion and tumor deposits were identified as independent prognostic markers for overall survival. Cox regression analysis showed that the tumor deposit positivity increased the risk of death of disease by 3.4-fold, whereas pericapsular invasion increased the risk of death by 2.2-fold.

Discussion About TDs in Head and Neck Carcinomas

Following the series by Violaris et al. and the two series performed by their group (Jose et al. 2004, 2007) in 2007, Jose et al. suggested that the importance of free tumor deposits should be appreciated due to very poor survival in cases with these lesions, in patients with head and neck carcinomas, and should be included in the pathology reports like the metastatic lymph nodes and metastatic lymph nodes with perinodal invasion. Furthermore the soft tissue tumor metastasis is not confined to the head and neck squamous cell carcinomas, but they may be observed in thyroid carcinoma-related metastasis. In medullary thyroid carcinoma cases, Gimm et al. identified disseminated tumor cells in neck dissection specimens in 15% of the patients in a series of 450 patients and suggested them to be a poor prognostic marker (Gimm et al. 2006). Jose et al. (2007) suggested that these were also lesions of the soft tumor deposit type. We have identified tumor deposits in the neck specimens of thyroid carcinoma cases (Figs. 8.20, 8.21, and 8.22).

Cutaneous squamous cell carcinomas are also among the cases which might present with neck tumor deposits. In 2012, Kelder et al. evaluated the tumor deposits in head and neck cutaneous squamous cell carcinomas. They found that the soft

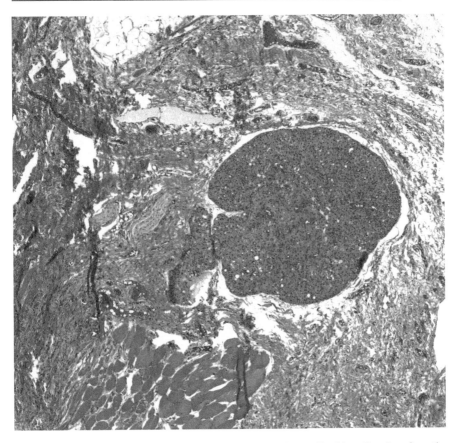

Fig. 8.20 Free tumor deposit arising from a follicular carcinoma Hurthle cell variant from the thyroid gland adjacent to neural structures (H&E, original magnification ×10)

tissue metastases have an adverse effect on survival compatible to multiple lymph node metastases. They suggested that adjuvant radiotherapy should be administered to all patients with STM, regardless of the diameter of the deposit, and pathology reports of head and neck SCC should include the presence, number, and size of STMs similar to the guidelines in melanoma and threshold for aggressive multimodal treatment should be considered in the presence of STM.

It should also be kept in mind that soft tissue tumor or free tumor deposits may be identified in clinically N0 cases. In a series of 63 cases and 96 neck dissection specimens of N0 cases by Coatesworth and MacLennan (2002), 19(30.2%) of the cases had lymph node metastasis and 12 had perinodal invasion, while 5(7.9%) patients had soft tissue deposits.

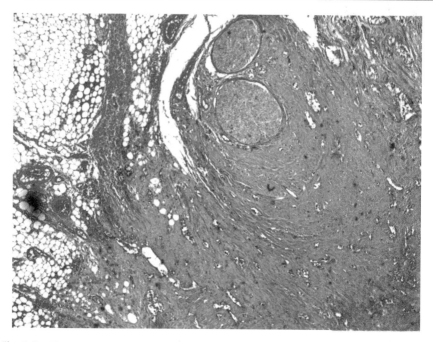

Fig. 8.21 Tumor deposit at the neck dissection material from a thyroid medullary carcinoma (H&E, original magnification ×10)

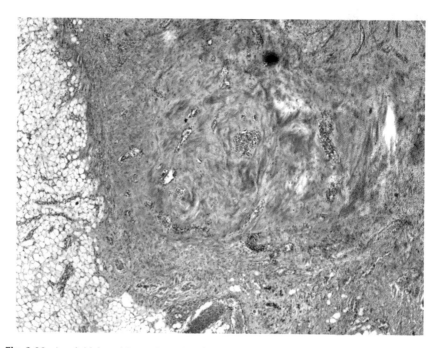

Fig. 8.22 Amyloid deposition at the tumor deposit at the neck dissection material from a thyroid medullary carcinoma (Congo Red, original magnification ×10)

References

Akman FC, Dag N, Ataman OU, Ecevit C, Ikiz AO, Arslan I, Sarioglu S, Ada E, Kinay M, Dokuz Eylul Head and Neck Tumour Group (DEHNTG). The impact of treatment center on the outcome of patients with laryngeal cancer treated with surgery and radiotherapy. Eur Arch Otorhinolaryngol. 2008;265(10):1245–55. https://doi.org/10.1007/s00405-008-0664-2; Epub 2008 Apr 5.

Cabanillas R, Secades P, Rodrigo JP, Astudillo A, Suárez C, Chiara MD. [Orthotopic murine model of head and neck squamous cell carcinoma]. Acta Otorrinolaringol Esp. 2005;56(3):89–95. Spanish.

Coatesworth AP, MacLennan K. Squamous cell carcinoma of the upper aerodigestive tract: the prevalence of microscopic extracapsular spread and soft tissue deposits in the clinically N0 neck. Head Neck. 2002;24(3):258–61.

College of American Pathologists. (2014). http://www.cap.org/apps/docs/committees/cancer/cancer_protocols/2013/Colon_13protocol_3300.pdf. Accessed 1 June 2017.

Demiral AN, Sarioglu S, Birlik B, Sen M, Kinay M. Prognostic significance of EGF receptor expression in early glottic cancer. Auris Nasus Larynx. 2004;31(4):417–24.

Goldstein NS, Turner JR. Pericolonic tumor deposits in patients with T3N+MO colon adenocarcinomas: markers of reduced disease free survival and intra-abdominal metastases and their implications for TNM classification. Cancer. 2000;88(10):2228–38.

El-Naggar AK, Takata T. Tumors of the oropharynx (base of tongue, tonsils, adenoids). In: El-Naggar AK, Ghan JKC, Grandis JF, Takata T, Slootweg PJ, editors. WHO classification of head and neck tumors. 4th ed. Lyon: IARC; 2017. p. 136–8.

Gimm O, Heyn V, Krause U, Sekulla C, Ukkat J, Dralle H. Prognostic significance of disseminated tumor cells in the connective tissue of patients with medullary thyroid carcinoma. World J Surg. 2006;30:847–52.

Jose J, Coatesworth AP, MacLennan K. Cervical metastases in upper aerodigestive tract squamous cell carcinoma: histopathologic analysis and reporting. Head Neck. 2003;25(3):194–7.

Jose J, Moor JW, Coatesworth AP, Johnston C, MacLennan K. Soft tissue deposits in neck dissections of patients with head and neck squamous cell carcinoma: prospective analysis of prevalence, survival, and its implications. Arch Otolaryngol Head Neck Surg. 2004;130(2):157–60.

Jose J, Ferlito A, Rodrigo JP, Devaney KO, Rinaldo A, MacLennan K. Soft tissue deposits from head and neck cancer: an under-recognised prognostic factor? J Laryngol Otol. 2007;121(12):1115–7.

Kelder W, Ebrahimi A, Forest VI, Gao K, Murali R, Clark JR. Cutaneous head and neck squamous cell carcinoma with regional metastases: the prognostic importance of soft tissue metastases and extranodal spread. Ann Surg Oncol. 2012;19(1):274–9. https://doi.org/10.1245/s10434-011-1986-7; Epub 2011 Aug 9.

Nur DA, Oguz C, Kemal, Ferhat E, Sülen S, Emel A, Münir K, Ann CS, Mehmet S. Prognostic factors in early glottic carcinoma implications for treatment. Tumori. 2005;91(2):182–7.

Sarioglu S, Acara C, Akman FC, Dag N, Ecevit C, Ikiz AO, Cetinayak OH, Ada E, for Dokuz Eylül Head and Neck Tumour Group (DEHNTG). Tumor budding as a prognostic marker in laryngeal carcinoma. Pathol Res Pract. 2010;206(2):88–92. https://doi.org/10.1016/j.prp.2009.09.006; Epub 2009 Dec 2.

Sarioglu S, Akbulut N, Iplikci S, Aydin B, Dogan E, Unlu M, Ellidokuz H, Ada E, Akman F, Ikiz AO. Tumor deposits in head and neck carcinomas. Head Neck. 2016;38(Suppl 1):E256–60. https://doi.org/10.1002/hed.23981; Epub 2015 Aug 21.

Sinha P, Lewis JS Jr, Kallogjeri D, Nussenbaum B, Haughey BH. Soft tissue metastasis in p16-positive oropharynx carcinoma: prevalence and association with distant metastasis. Oral Oncol. 2015;51(8):778–86. https://doi.org/10.1016/j.oraloncology.2015.05.004; Epub 2015 May 29.

Slootweg PJ, Chan JKC, Stelow EB, Thompson LDR. Tumors of the nasal cavity, paranasal sinuses and skull base. In: El-Naggar AK, Ghan JKC, Grandis JF, Takata T, Slootweg PJ, editors. WHO classification of head and neck tumors. 4th ed. Lyon: IARC; 2017. p. 14–27.

Slootweg PJ, Grandis JR. Tumors of the hypopharynx, larynx and parapharyngeal spaces. In: El-Naggar AK, Ghan JKC, Grandis JF, Takata T, Slootweg PJ, editors. WHO classification of head and neck tumors. 4th ed. Lyon: IARC; 2017. p. 81–90.

Ueno H, Mochizuki H, Hashiguchi Y, Ishiguro M, Miyoshi M, Kajiwara Y, Sato T, Shimazaki H, Hase K. Extramural cancer deposits without nodal structure in colorectal cancer: optimal categorization for prognostic staging. Am J Clin Pathol. 2007;127(2):287–94.

Unlu M, Cetinayak HO, Onder D, Ecevit C, Akman F, Ikız AÖ, Ada E, Karacali B, Sarioglu S. The prognostic value of tumor-stroma proportion in laryngeal squamous cell carcinoma. Turk Patoloji Derg. 2013;29(1):27–35. https://doi.org/10.5146/tjpath.2013.01144.

Violaris NS, O'Neil D, Helliwell TR, Caslin AW, Roland NJ, Jones AS. Soft tissue cervical metastases of squamous carcinoma of the head and neck. Clin Otolaryngol Allied Sci. 1994;19(5):394–9.

Tumor Deposits in Breast Carcinomas

9

Breast carcinomas are the most common carcinomas in women. Early diagnosis and recent treatment methods improved the survival in the last decades; however, they are still a major health problem.

Classification of Breast Carcinomas

The breast carcinoma cases may be divided into two categories as in situ and invasive types. According to the WHO 2012 classification, invasive carcinoma of no special type (ductal, not otherwise specified) and invasive lobular breast carcinomas are the most frequent types. Each of the other types of carcinomas makes up less than 5% or even 1% of the cases. As the name implies, invasive carcinoma of no special type (ductal, not otherwise specified) is a diagnosis of exclusion. In different series, the incidence of this type of carcinoma ranges between 40 and 75%, probably related to the strictness of the criteria for inclusion among special types (Fig. 9.1). Invasive lobular carcinoma makes up 5–15% of the cases (Figs. 9.2, 9.3, and 9.4).

The histopathological grading of the breast carcinomas is an important feature of the histopathological evaluation of the breast carcinoma cases and should be applied for all invasive carcinoma cases. The method for invasive breast carcinoma grading is Nottingham combined histologic grade (Elston-Ellis modification of Scarff-Bloom-Richardson grading system) (Elston and Ellis 1991) and should be used for pathology reporting. In this system, the amount of tubule formation, nuclear pleomorphism, and mitotic count are scored as 1, 2, or 3. The addition of these three scores gives the overall grade score as follows:

Grade I: 3, 4, and 5
Grade II: 6 and 7
Grade III: 8 and 9

© Springer International Publishing AG 2018
S. Sarioglu, *Tumor Deposits*, https://doi.org/10.1007/978-3-319-68582-3_9

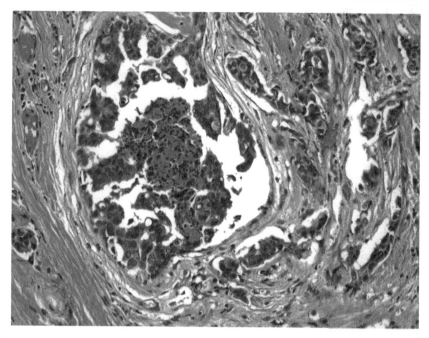

Fig. 9.1 Comedo type of necrosis in an invasive ductal carcinoma (H&E, original magnification ×40) (Courtesy of Associate Prof. Merih Guray Durak, Dokuz Eylul University, Izmir, Turkey)

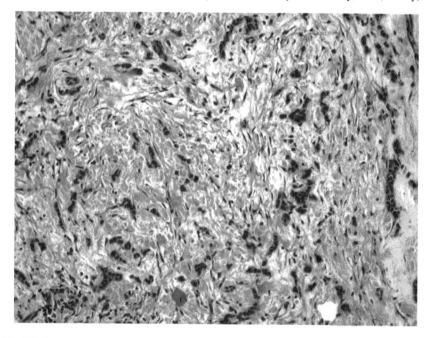

Fig. 9.2 Invasive tumor characterized by proliferation of small cells arranged in single-cell linear cords; invasive lobular carcinoma (H&E, original magnification ×20) (Courtesy of Associate Prof. Merih Guray Durak, Dokuz Eylul University, Izmir, Turkey)

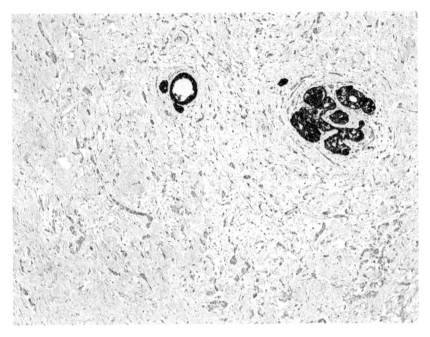

Fig. 9.3 Loss of E-cadherin expression in invasive lobular carcinoma (IHC E-cadherin, original magnification ×20) (Courtesy of Associate Prof. Merih Guray Durak, Dokuz Eylul University, Izmir, Turkey)

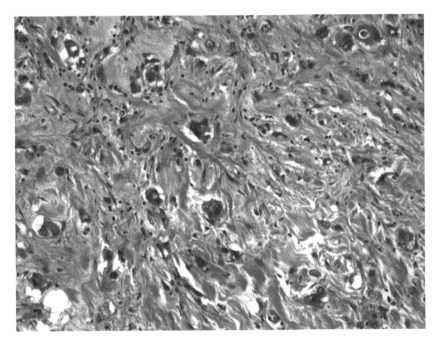

Fig. 9.4 Pleomorphic lobular carcinoma; marked nuclear atypia is the typical feature of these cases, while the pattern of invasion is similar to a classical lobular carcinoma case (H&E, original magnification ×20) (Courtesy of Associate Prof. Merih Guray Durak, Dokuz Eylul University, Izmir, Turkey)

If only microinvasive pattern is observed, histological grading is not applied.

The other rare patterns make up small proportions of this disease. The cases and their frequencies among all breast carcinoma cases and some microscopic images may be listed as follows: invasive micropapillary carcinoma (0.9–2%) (Fig. 9.5), mucinous carcinoma (2%) (Fig. 9.6), tubular carcinoma (2%), invasive cribriform carcinoma (<%1) (Fig. 9.7), invasive papillary carcinoma (<1%) (Fig. 9.8), medullary carcinoma (<1%), metaplastic carcinoma (0.2–5%), low-grade adenosquamous carcinoma (<1%), squamous cell carcinoma (<1%), salivary gland/skin adnexal type including adenoid cystic carcinoma (<0.1%), mucoepidermoid (0.3%), invasive carcinoma with apocrine features such as apocrine differentiation (NST, tubular, micropapillary, medullary) (Fig. 9.9), invasive carcinoma with clear-cell (glycogen-rich) features (1–3%), invasive carcinoma with neuroendocrine features (<1%), invasive carcinoma with signet-ring cell features (<1%), and secretory carcinoma (<0.15%) (CAP 2017; Lakhani et al. 2012).

The hormonal receptor status of the breast carcinomas is important both as prognostic and predictive factors. Estrogen receptor (ER) expression is positive in 80%, and progesterone receptor (PR) is positive in 40% of the cases. Therapies targeting the blockage of ER have been used for treatment, and these are more successful in cases with PR positivity which reflects the intact and functioning ER pathway (Arpino et al. 2005) (Figs. 9.10 and 9.11).

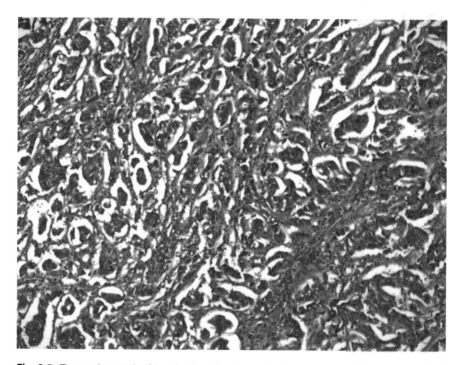

Fig. 9.5 Tumor characterized by clusters of cells growing in empty stromal spaces, devoid of fibrovascular core. At first, each cluster seems like lymphatic invasion. Inside-out location of the glandular cells is typical for these cases (H&E, original magnification ×20) (Courtesy of Associate Prof. Merih Guray Durak, Dokuz Eylul University, Izmir, Turkey)

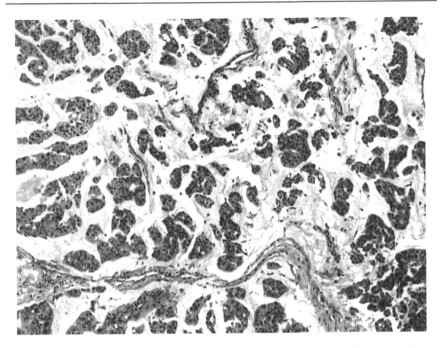

Fig. 9.6 Mucinous carcinoma, tumor cells swimming in extracellular mucin pools (H&E, original magnification ×20) (Courtesy of Associate Prof. Merih Guray Durak, Dokuz Eylul University, Izmir, Turkey)

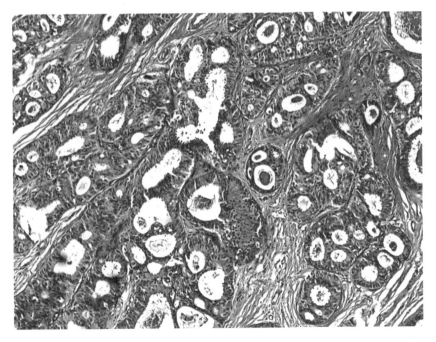

Fig. 9.7 Cribriform carcinoma; the pattern resembles adenoid cystic carcinoma, but there is no myoepithelial differentiation. Pure form of this rare tumor is associated with good prognosis (H&E, original magnification ×20) (Courtesy of Associate Prof. Merih Guray Durak, Dokuz Eylul University, Izmir, Turkey)

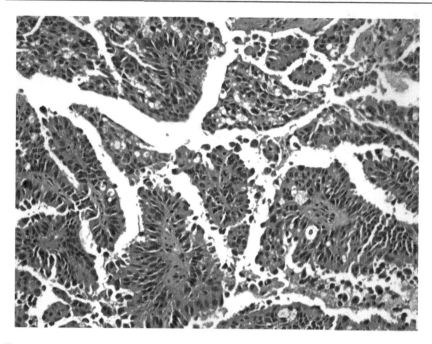

Fig. 9.8 Invasive papillary carcinoma is a very rare tumor with crowded papillary structures made up of malignant cells (H&E, original magnification ×20) (Courtesy of Associate Prof. Merih Guray Durak, Dokuz Eylul University, Izmir, Turkey)

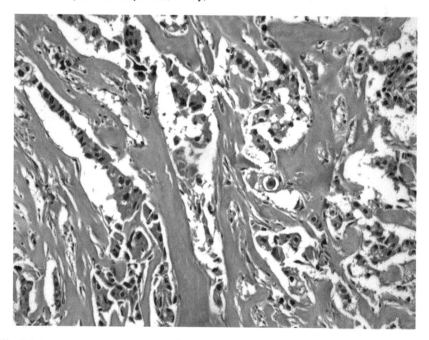

Fig. 9.9 Invasive carcinoma with apocrine features (H&E, original magnification ×20) (Courtesy of Associate Prof. Merih Guray Durak, Dokuz Eylul University, Izmir, Turkey)

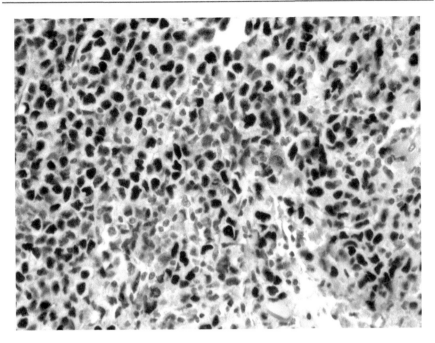

Fig. 9.10 All the nuclei are strongly stained in a breast carcinoma without tubular architecture; tubule formation score: 3 (IHC, estrogen receptor, original magnification ×20) (Courtesy of Associate Prof. Merih Guray Durak, Dokuz Eylul University, Izmir, Turkey)

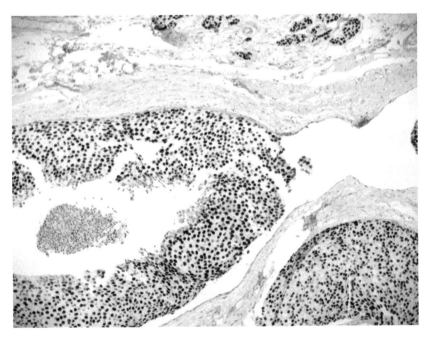

Fig. 9.11 A breast carcinoma with intraductal component, strong nuclear positivity (IHC, progesterone receptor, original magnification ×20) (Courtesy of Associate Prof. Merih Guray Durak, Dokuz Eylul University, Izmir, Turkey)

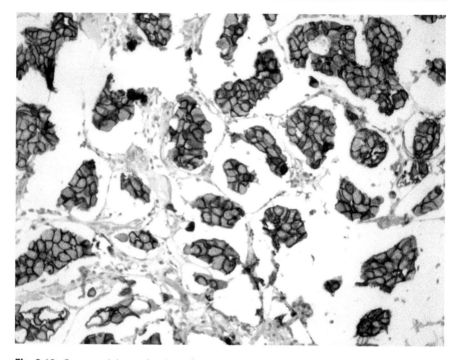

Fig. 9.12 Strong staining at the circumferential cytoplasmic membranes of the breast carcinoma cells; c-erbB2 expression (+++). In this case, in situ hybridization for HER2 gene amplification is not necessary, as (+++) positive IHC staining is diagnostic (IHC, c-erbB2, original magnification ×20) (Courtesy of Associate Prof. Merih Guray Durak, Dokuz Eylul University, Izmir, Turkey)

HER2 amplification is associated with poor prognosis, and specific antibodies against these receptors are treatment options for patients with this type of amplification (Tong et al. 2017). HER2 amplification can be detected by immunohistochemistry methods, cytoplasmic, membranous, strong, and circumferential staining; (+++) staining is diagnostic for this amplification (Fig. 9.12). However, if (++) staining is observed, in situ hybridization should be applied for detection.

Molecular subtypes of breast carcinomas were classified as follows:

Luminal A: Grade I and II, low ki-67 expression, and ER+/HER2- are the features of this group. Invasive carcinoma not specified and classic lobular, tubular, cribriform, mucinous, and neuroendocrine carcinomas may be seen. *PIK3CA*, *MAP3KI*, *GATA3*, and *FOXA1* mutations, *ESR1* and *XBP1* high expression, quiet genomes, gain of 1q and 8q, and loss of 8p and 16q are frequent.

Luminal B: Grade II and III, high ki-67 expression, and ER+ or —/HER2+ or — are the features of this group. Invasive carcinoma not specified and micropapillary carcinoma are the histological types. *TP53* and *PIK3CA* mutations, *cyclin D1* and *MDM2* amplification, *ATM* loss, enhanced genomic instability, and focal amplifications are frequent.

HER2: Grade II and III, high ki-67 expression, and ER+ or —/HER2+ are the features of this group. Invasive carcinoma not specified and apocrine and pleomorphic lobular carcinomas may be seen. *HER2* and *cyclin D1* amplifications; *TP53*, *PIK3CA*, and *APOBEC* mutations; and *FGFR4* and *EGFR* high expression are frequent.

Basal-Like: Grade III, high ki-67 expression, and ER-/HER2- are the features of this group. Invasive carcinoma not specified and medullary, metaplastic, adenoid cystic, and secretory carcinomas may be seen in this group. *TP53* mutations, *RB1* and *BRCA1* loss, high expression of DNA repair proteins, *FOXM1* activation, high genomic instability, and focal amplifications are frequent. t(12;15)(p13;q25) ETV6-NTRK3 fusion gene is very frequent in secretory carcinoma, and the t(6;9)(q22–23;p23–24) MYB-NFIB fusion gene is frequent in adenoid cystic carcinoma (Curtis et al. 2012; Vuong et al. 2014).

The triple-negative group (ER(−)/PR(−)/HER2(−)) cases include basal-like (CK5/6 + and/or EGFR+) and normal-like breast carcinomas (CK5/6- and/or EGFR-) (Badowska-Kozakiewicz and Budzik 2016) with different prognostic features and different treatment options.

Many morphological features of the breast carcinomas and molecular changes were investigated in a large series of breast carcinomas (Heng et al. 2017).

Prognosis and Tumor Deposits in Breast Carcinomas

Tumor diameter, grade, lymphovascular invasion, lymph node, ER/PR, and HER2 status are the most important factors in decision making for the treatment of the breast carcinomas; however, many gene signature studies are being carried out (van de Vijver 2014).

Lymph node metastasis is a poor prognostic marker for breast carcinoma patients as in many types of carcinomas. High mitotic indexes, tumors larger than 2 cm, and angiolymphatic invasion are associated with increased axillary metastasis (Aquino et al. 2017). The identification of tumor metastasis in sentinel lymph nodes is important for the planning of the extent of the surgical procedure and has been used nearly for 30 years now. The diameter of the metastatic tumor at the lymph nodes is also a prognostic marker (Meattini et al. 2014). The factors that predict non-sentinel lymph node metastasis include the area percent of sentinel node occupied by tumor and the number of sentinel nodes removed (Durak MG et al. 2011). Extranodal invasion is a poor prognostic factor in breast carcinoma cases. In the series of breast carcinoma and lymph node metastasis cases by Külahcı et al. (2017), 34.58% of the cases had extranodal invasion. In the meta-analysis by Nottegar et al. (2016), about the prognostic value of extranodal invasion, five articles were selected, and of the 624 cases, 26.12% had extranodal invasion. Extranodal invasion was associated with a higher risk of both mortality (OR = 2.51) and recurrence of disease (OR = 2.07).

Lymph node metastasis and extranodal invasion are poor prognostic markers in many types of carcinomas including esophageal, colon, head and neck, as well as gastric carcinomas. However, in these cases, free tumor deposits are also identified as poor prognostic factors.

Free tumor deposits are most widely recognized and included in the TNM classifications of the colorectal carcinoma cases. These lesions are also named as extranodal metastasis or satellites, and they are described as "tumor nodules with regular or irregular contours, located away from the primary tumor mass, but within the lymphatic draining area, devoid of the morphological features of a lymph node" in the colorectal CAP templates for tumor reporting (CAP 2013).

In the series of Al Sahaf et al. (2011), perinodal invasion and TD were identified as prognostic markers in stage II and III colon carcinomas. They found lymph node ratio, extracapsular lymph node extension, and adjuvant chemotherapy as independent prognostic markers of both disease-free survival and overall survival. The survival of TD-positive cases at 5 years was 11%, while perinodal invasion was associated with 33% 5-year survival. Perinodal invasion is a poor prognostic marker in esophageal carcinomas as well as the tumor deposits at the gastroesophageal junction carcinoma cases (Metzger et al. 2009; Zhang et al. 2013). In salivary gland tumors, Walvekar et al. (2011) identified extracapsular spread as an independent predictor of disease-free survival in a series of 115 cases. In our series of head and neck carcinomas, tumor deposit positivity and pericapsular invasion increased the disease-related death by 3.4-fold and 2.2-fold, respectively (Sarioglu et al. 2016). Although many prognostic features like lymph node metastasis and perinodal invasion were evaluated and identified as poor prognostic markers in breast carcinomas, tumor deposits seem to be neglected. In fact these are easily detected in axillary dissection materials and accepted as lymph node metastasis.

Although there are no series evaluating the incidence and prognostic value of tumor deposits in breast carcinomas, it is easy to present microscopic images of such lesions from breast carcinoma cases. Such lesions should be differentiated from metastatic lymph nodes and extranodal invasion as in carcinomas of different organs like the colorectal and head and neck carcinoma cases (Figs. 9.13, 9.14, 9.15, 9.16, 9.17, and 9.18).

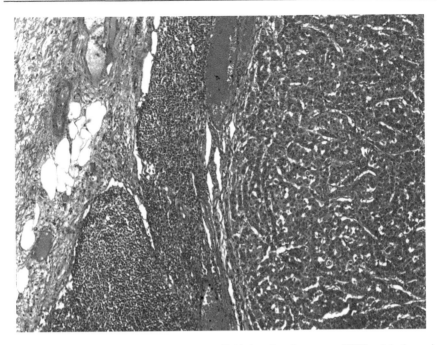

Fig. 9.13 Metastatic lymph node with easily, identifiable lymph node structure (H&E, original magnification ×20) (Courtesy of Associate Prof. Merih Guray Durak, Dokuz Eylul University, Izmir, Turkey)

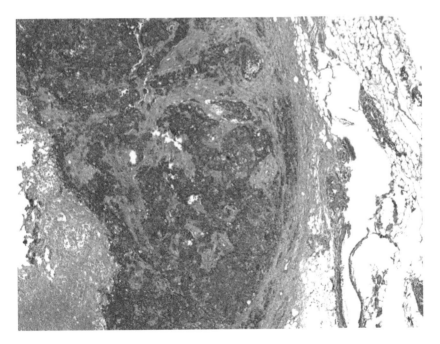

Fig. 9.14 A free tumor deposit without any identifiable lymph node structure. The regular contours of such deposits may cause concern of the pathologists about wrong diagnosis of a metastatic lymph node (H&E, original magnification ×20) (Courtesy of Associate Prof. Merih Guray Durak, Dokuz Eylul University, Izmir, Turkey)

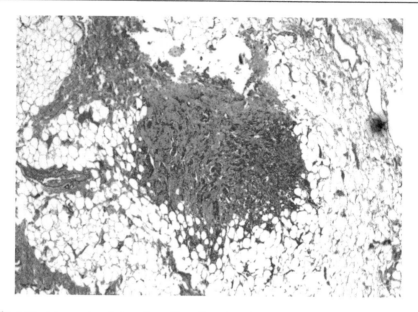

Fig. 9.15 A tumor deposit from the axillary dissection of a breast carcinoma with irregular contours. This lesion would be classified as a tumor deposit if it was dissected from a colectomy specimen (H&E, original magnification ×10) (Courtesy of Associate Prof. Merih Guray Durak, Dokuz Eylul University, Izmir, Turkey)

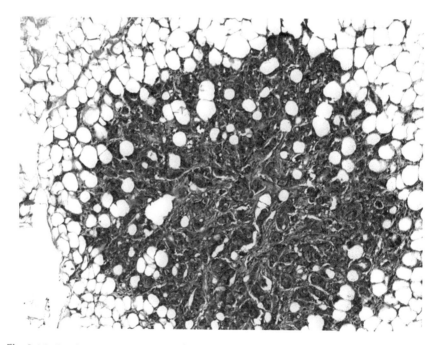

Fig. 9.16 Another tumor deposit from the axillary dissection of a breast carcinoma with irregular contours (H&E, original magnification ×20) (Courtesy of Associate Prof. Merih Guray Durak, Dokuz Eylul University, Izmir, Turkey)

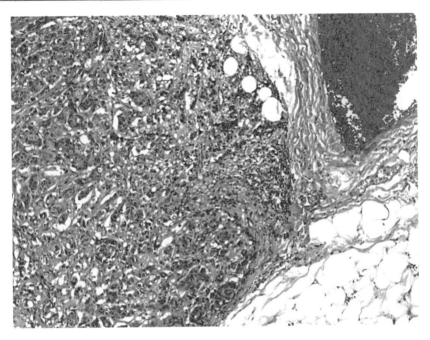

Fig. 9.17 A perivascular tumor deposit with regular contours (H&E, original magnification ×10) (Courtesy of Associate Prof. Merih Guray Durak, Dokuz Eylul University, Izmir, Turkey)

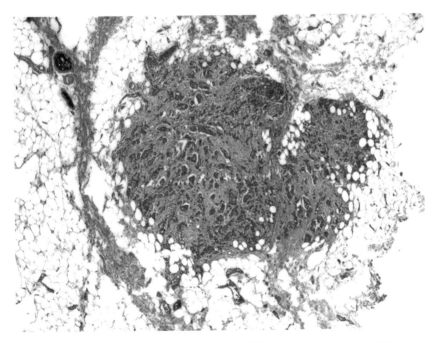

Fig. 9.18 Desmoplastic reaction at a tumor deposit (H&E, original magnification ×10) (Courtesy of Associate Prof. Merih Guray Durak, Dokuz Eylul University, Izmir, Turkey)

Conclusions

Breast carcinomas are among the most frequent carcinomas, and much research has been focused on the prognostic and predictive factors of these tumors resulting in better survival. However, recognizing mechanisms resulting in poor survival and presenting treatment options are of utmost importance. Extravascular perineural and perivascular spread seem to be important in the progression of tumor deposits, and neglecting these mechanisms of spread may result in undertreatment of patients. The extensive studies about breast carcinomas should include the tumor deposits.

References

Al Sahaf O, Myers E, Jawad M, Browne TJ, Winter DC, Redmond HP. The prognostic significance of extramural deposits and extracapsular lymph node invasion in colon cancer. Dis Colon Rectum. 2011;54(8):982–8. https://doi.org/10.1097/DCR.0b013e31821c4944.

Aquino RGF, Vasques PHD, Cavalcante DIM, Oliveira ALS, Oliveira BMK, Pinheiro LGP. Invasive ductal carcinoma: relationship between pathological characteristics and the presence of axillary metastasis in 220 cases. Rev Col Bras Cir. 2017;44(2):163–70. https://doi.org/10.1590/0100-69912017002010. English, Portuguese.

Arpino G, Weiss H, Lee AV, Schiff R, De Placido S, Osborne CK, Elledge RM. Estrogen receptor-positive, progesterone receptor-negative breast cancer: association with growth factor receptor expression and tamoxifen resistance. J Natl Cancer Inst. 2005;97:1254–61. https://doi.org/10.1093/jnci/dji249.

Badowska-Kozakiewicz AM, Budzik MP. Immunohistochemical characteristics of basal-like breast cancer. Contemp Oncol (Pozn). 2016;20(6):436–43. https://doi.org/10.5114/wo.2016.56938. Epub 2017 Jan 12. Review.

CAP. (2013). http://www.cap.org/ShowProperty?nodePath=/UCMCon/Contribution%20Folders/WebContent/pdf/colon-13protocol-3300.pdf. Accessed 24 April 2017.

CAP. (2017). http://www.cap.org/ShowProperty?nodePath=/UCMCon/Contribution%20Folders/WebContent/pdf/cp-breast-invasive-17protocol-4000.pdf. Accessed 13 Aug 2017.

Curtis C, Shah SP, Chin SF, Turashvili G, Rueda OM, Dunning MJ, Speed D, Lynch AG, Samarajiwa S, Yuan Y, Gräf S, Ha G, Haffari G, Bashashati A, Russell R, McKinney S, METABRIC Group, Langerød A, Green A, Provenzano E, Wishart G, Pinder S, Watson P, Markowetz F, Murphy L, Ellis I, Purushotham A, Børresen-Dale AL, Brenton JD, Tavaré S, Caldas C, Aparicio S. The genomic and transcriptomic architecture of 2,000 breast tumours reveals novel subgroups. Nature. 2012;486(7403):346–52. https://doi.org/10.1038/nature10983.

Durak MG, Akansu B, Akin MM, Sevınç AI, Koçdor MA, Saydam S, Harmancioğlu O, Ellıdokuz H, Bekış R, Canda T. Factors predicting non-sentinel lymph node involvement in sentinel node positive breast carcinoma. Turk Patoloji Derg. 2011;27(3):189–95. https://doi.org/10.5146/tjpath.2011.01074.

Elston CW, Ellis IO. Pathological prognostic factors in breast cancer. I. The value of histological grade in breast cancer: experience from a large study with long-term follow-up. Histopathology. 1991;19(5):403–10.

Heng YJ, Lester SC, Tse GM, Factor RE, Allison KH, Collins LC, Chen YY, Jensen KC, Johnson NB, Jeong JC, Punjabi R, Shin SJ, Singh K, Krings G, Eberhard DA, Tan PH, Korski K, Waldman FM, Gutman DA, Sanders M, Reis-Filho JS, Flanagan SR, Gendoo DM, Chen GM, Haibe-Kains B, Ciriello G, Hoadley KA, Perou CM, Beck AH. The molecular basis of breast cancer pathological phenotypes. J Pathol. 2017;241(3):375–91. https://doi.org/10.1002/path.4847; Epub 2016 Dec 29.

Külahcı Ö, Esen HH, Asut E, Güngör S. Association of ICAM-1, VCAM-1, CYCLIN D1 and cathepsin D with clinicopathological parameters in breast carcinoma; an immunohistochemical study. J Breast Health (2013). 2017;13(1):5–9. https://doi.org/10.5152/tjbh.2016.3142; eCollection 2017 Jan.

Lakhani SR, Ellis IO, Schnitt SJ, Tan PH, van de Vijver MJ, editors. WHO classification of breast tumors. Lyon: IARC; 2012.

Meattini I, Desideri I, Saieva C, Francolini G, Scotti V, Bonomo P, Greto D, Mangoni M, Nori J, Orzalesi L, Fambrini M, Bianchi S, Livi L. Impact of sentinel node tumor burden on outcome of invasive breast cancer patients. Eur J Surg Oncol. 2014;40(10):1195–202. https://doi.org/10.1016/j.ejso.2014.08.471; Epub 2014 Aug 20.

Metzger R, Drebber U, Baldus SE, Mönig SP, Hölscher AH, Bollschweiler E. Extracapsular lymph node involvement differs between squamous cell and adenocarcinoma of the esophagus. Ann Surg Oncol. 2009;16(2):447–53. https://doi.org/10.1245/s10434-008-0248-9; Epub 2008 Nov 27.

Nottegar A, Veronese N, Senthil M, Roumen RM, Stubbs B, Choi AH, Verheuvel NC, Solmi M, Pea A, Capelli P, Fassan M, Sergi G, Manzato E, Maruzzo M, Bagante F, Koç M, Eryilmaz MA, Bria E, Carbognin L, Bonetti F, Barbareschi M, Luchini C. Extra-nodal extension of sentinel lymph node metastasis is a marker of poor prognosis in breast cancer patients: a systematic review and an exploratory meta-analysis. Eur J Surg Oncol. 2016;42(7):919–25. https://doi.org/10.1016/j.ejso.2016.02.259; Epub 2016 Mar 10. Review.

Sarioglu S, Akbulut N, Iplikci S, Aydin B, Dogan E, Unlu M, Ellidokuz H, Ada E, Akman F, Ikiz AO. Tumor deposits in head and neck carcinomas. Head Neck. 2016;38(Suppl 1):E256–60. https://doi.org/10.1002/hed.23981; Epub 2015 Aug 21.

Tong ZJ, Shi NY, Zhang ZJ, Yuan XD, Hong XM. Expression and prognostic value of HER-2/neu in primary breast cancer with sentinel lymph node metastasis. Biosci Rep. 2017;37(4). https://doi.org/10.1042/BSR20170121; Print 2017 Aug 31.

van de Vijver MJ. Molecular tests as prognostic factors in breast cancer. Virchows Arch. 2014;464:283–91. https://doi.org/10.1007/s00428014-1539-0.

Vuong D, Simpson PT, Green B, Cummings MC, Lakhani SR. Molecular classification of breast cancer. Virchows Arch. 2014;465(1):1–14. https://doi.org/10.1007/s00428-014-1593-7; Epub 2014 May 31.

Walvekar RR, Andrade Filho PA, Seethala RR, Gooding WE, Heron DE, Johnson JT, Ferris RL. Clinicopathologic features as stronger prognostic factors than histology or grade in risk stratification of primary parotid malignancies. Head Neck. 2011;33(2):225–31.

Zhang HD, Tang P, Duan XF, Chen CG, Ma Z, Gao YY, Zhang H, Yu ZT. Extranodal metastasis is a powerful prognostic factor in patients with adenocarcinoma of the esophagogastric junction. J Surg Oncol. 2013;108(8):542–9.

Index

© Springer International Publishing AG 2018   187
S. Sarioglu, *Tumor Deposits*, https://doi.org/10.1007/978-3-319-68582-3